Occupational Therapy
for the
Energy Deficient Patient

The *Occupational Therapy in Health Care* series,
Florence S. Cromwell, Editor

- *The Changing Roles of Occupational Therapists in the 1980s*
- *Occupational Therapy Assessment as the Keystone to Treatment Planning*
- *Occupational Therapy and the Patient With Pain*
- *Occupational Therapy Strategies and Adaptations for Independent Daily Living*
- *The Roles of Occupational Therapists in Continuity of Care*
- *Private Practice in Occupational Therapy*
- *Occupational Therapy and Adolescents with Disability*
- *Work-Related Programs in Occupational Therapy*
- *Occupational Therapy for the Energy Deficient Patient*

Occupational Therapy for the Energy Deficient Patient

Florence S. Cromwell
Editor

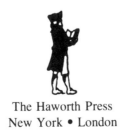

The Haworth Press
New York • London

Occupational Therapy for the Energy Deficient Patient has also been published as *Occupational Therapy in Health Care,* Volume 3, Number 1, Spring 1986.

The Haworth Press, Inc., 28 East 22 Street, New York, NY 10010-6194
EUROSPAN/Haworth, 3 Henrietta Street, WC2E 8LU England

Library of Congress Cataloging in Publication Data
  Main entry under title:

Occupational therapy for the energy deficient patient.

   Published also as: Occupational therapy in health care, v. 3, no. 1, spring 1986.
   Includes bibliographies.
      1. Occupational therapy. 2. Fatigue—Treatment. I. Cromwell, Florence S. [DNLM:
1. Occupational Therapy. W1 OC601H v.3 no.1 / WB 555 0144]
   RM735.034   1986   615.8'5152   85-27277
   ISBN 0-86656-550-7
   ISBN 0-86656-551-5 (pbk.)

Occupational Therapy for the Energy Deficient Patient

Occupational Therapy in Health Care
Volume 3, Number 1

CONTENTS

SOMETHING NEW AND USEFUL . . .

Occupational Therapy
for the
Energy Deficient Patient

FROM THE EDITOR'S DESK

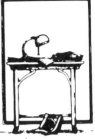

The choice of 'low energy' as the focus for this issue of *OTHC* seemed a very natural one to offer to occupational therapist readers. After all, *activity* is the centerpiece of the profession's philosophy of health preservation. Further, *engagement* of patients in purposeful activity is the linchpin in the implementation of the profession's major theories of treatment. Given the range of problems and the severity of disability of the persons occupational therapists serve, it follows that *energy* considerations, both biological and psychological, are often critical to the effectiveness of treatment regardless of how well we plan. Energy deficits are 'givens' in so many of the disabilities common in the practice rosters of occupational therapy clinics. Low energy often literally prevents effective performance of activities of daily living in the broadest sense. So, the low energy or energy deficient patient is an ongoing concern for practitioners. This issue of *OTHC* hopes to draw renewed attention to this consequence of many illnesses and accidents and offer some ideas that occupational therapists can and do use for confronting and overcoming low energy as a barrier to satisfying independent daily living.

Parent's introductory paper provides the historical perspective on the profession's ongoing attention to energy as the critical element in daily activity and appropriately speaks of energy as 'the illusive factor' in treatment planning. Her presentation provides important understandings, principally of biological energy, and she suggests many ways in which therapists can address energy deficiencies in their patients. Her bibliography is also a rich resource on the sub-

1

ject. Rosenbusch, on the other hand, introduces a concept undoubtedly new as a treatment strategy to many readers' thinking—psychic energy, and suggests greater understanding of its potentials as an untapped resource in working with severely disabled people. Miyake and his cohorts remind us of the 'energy' problems of many in the psychiatric population by addressing depression and the difficulties of engaging persons so affected. His proposals for imparting purpose in treatment suggest that both biological and psychic energy are involved in working with persons with depression.

We all readily recognize low energy resources as characteristics of persons with stroke, arthritis, high level spinal cord injury as well as in persons with severe heart and lung disease and other debilitating illnesses. However, Washburn turns our attention to what may seem obvious concepts of occupational therapy but now applied to planning environments for the elderly for whom declining energy is an ever present factor. She suggests that given the demographics in our country, the participation of occupational therapists in planning living spaces for the growing numbers of older persons is urgently needed to assure *healthy* aging.

Clarke in the same vein, draws our attention to low energy or scarce energy as an important consideration in determining how one approaches preparation for lifelong independence for children with multiple limb deficiencies. Too often occupational therapists, it would seem, have planned for learned behaviors and uses of equipment in ADL as the focus of treatment for severely disabled persons and only *intuitively* have been attentive to energy considerations. Clarke's illustrative case emphasizes, from the patient's point of view, how critical energy is in daily planning despite having all the skills one needs to be independent—a forceful lesson for us in planning for both children and adult patients.

Since patients with heart and lung disease are so numerous in many treatment programs and present such obvious energy considerations to therapists, four papers are included addressing treatment approaches to these persons. Walsh provides a comprehensive program overview from a center known historically for its concern for persons with lung disease. Phillips presents an evaluation strategy that can be useful in any setting where energy awareness is a focus. Similarly, Haid provides a model for monitored task evaluation as a tool to use as part of a comprehensive program of cardiac care, while Bird and Phelps place emphasis, in their paper, on the psychological components of cardiac programming as important elements of energy use.

There are admittedly many treatment programs created by occupational therapists that confront difficulties in performance of activities of daily living and even specifically the need for attention to energy as the facilitator of successful performance. We could have highlighted many more examples in this issue. Marvelous strategies and tools have been developed and used to help patients compensate for deficiencies—from reach to time management, from coordination to decision making. But each time we learn of another program, or another treatment strategy, another link is forged in the profession's activity theory. The exchange offered by the few papers in this issue will hopefully contribute to that process.

But for all the strategies devised and used by therapists, engagement of patients in activity programs is the final objective to improve/enhance their daily living. If one has limited energy he obviously must be guided in learning *how* to do things more easily, but then to *choose* the things to do in daily life that give him most satisfaction. Thus he spends his energy for what is important to him. Our feature, *Practice Watch,* by Lindheim presents a vignette of a lady who has, as a more or less typical survivor of stroke, learned to make those choices and thereby has made a remarkable adjustment to disability. She has adapted her life style to her diminished functional level largely because of her own determination and, could we say, her psychic energy? She has indeed capitalized on *will* as the energy to fuel her daily activity in those things she finds it important to do. She offers therapists therby an enticing thought. How can we energize the will of patients?

The other feature, *Something New and Different,* is indeed that, a game which therapists and others working with the elder population and their caregivers will find intriguing and useful. It is included in this issue both because older persons are part of our focus as we address energy, and because, as Lindheim enunciates in her account of her grandmother's recovery, unless we can be sensitive to attitudes and values of our patients we may find all our energies spent for naught.

Looking ahead, the next issue of *OTHC* will be directed to the role of occupational therapy in eating/feeding/dining activities. Watch for it as we try to highlight occupational therapists as the *key* persons in this aspect of rehabilitation programming.

Looking back over Volume II, I realize it is time to acknowledge again the contributions made by the Editorial Board for their many hours of volunteer labor in which they offered significant help to our writers and to this editor. Also, in the volume a number of special, 'expert' reviewers were called upon and a new group of book reviewers were added. All of these people helped your editor enormously, and I would like to acknowledge them:

Stephanie Day   Jan Liptak
Mary M. Evert   Helen E. Lowe
Jane T. Herrick   Kathy Reynolds-Lynch
Janith Hurff   Karen Schultz
Jerry A. Johnson   Lynn Yasuda
Kristin L. Keenan

Finally, I wish to say a special thanks to six members of the original Editorial Board who are completing two year terms and wish to 'retire' to other activities, or to just 'special' reviewing jobs. They are:

Tone F. Blechert, COTA,   Susan Livingston Davis, OTR
    ROH   Anne Larson, OT(C)
Pamela H. Brown, COTA   Janet C. Stone, OTR
Betty Cox, COTA, ROH

Beginning in Volume III, new persons will assume their responsibilities.

Florence S. Cromwell
Editor

Energy: The Illusive Factor in Daily Activity

Lillian Hoyle Parent, MA, OTR, FAOTA

ABSTRACT. Historically occupational therapists have planned treatment programs requiring activity involving different and diverse amounts of energy use by patients. Also, many energy saving methods and devices, now commonly applied by therapists, were developed empirically to make activities possible for paralyzed patients. For the energy deficient patient physiological concepts of energy may not apply because both psychological and sociological factors may influence how individuals convert food to energy for maintenance of homeostasis and musculoskeletal activity. Energy conservation measures, identified with occupational therapy, may be supplemented with Brief, Isometric, Maximal Exercise (BRIME) to enhance energy reserves, and reflex mechanisms may also be used to facilitate movement for the energy deficient person. The older person with low energy but without serious medical problems may need thorough investigation of life style and environment in order to plan appropriate occupational therapy intervention.

Energy is a physiological concept about which researchers in that field admit there are many aspects that remain little known or studied.[1] Occupational therapists have long treated those patients whose strength was diminished through neuromuscular disease. The relationship of approaches to patients with those problems to present concepts regarding the 'energy deficient' patient will be described. The puzzle that energy use presents to researchers in physiology is discussed. The use of BRIME exercise and of reflex movement patterns are suggested as methods to teach patients ways of conserving energy.

Lillian Hoyle Parent, Coordinator Education and Research, Department of Occupational Therapy, University of Texas Medical Branch, Galveston, TX 77550.

This article appears jointly in *Occupational Therapy for the Energy Deficient Patient* (The Haworth Press, 1986), and *Occupational Therapy in Health Care*, Volume 3, Number 1 (Spring 1986).

5

HISTORY

Occupational therapists have often found it necessary to balance action and inaction in planning patient activities. For example, the goal was to find activities to help calm the chronically disturbed mental patient versus stimulating the depressed and reclusive patient to more activity and awareness.[2] Individuals with tuberculosis were placed on a regimen that reduced their activity levels to a minimum while at the same time various methods were used to maintain mental well-being so that rest and time could overcome the bacterial invasion that had debilitated them. Occupational therapists working with the tuberculous patient became skilled in planning treatment programs of graded activity, depending upon the patient's stage of recovery and the amount of activity allowed for that stage.[3] Judgement about the strenuousness of the activity chosen was intuitive and it was not until the 1950's that knowledge of the amounts of energy, either metabolic equivalent or cardiac output, was published for many activities of daily living, occupational therapy activities and work and leisure activities.[4,5,6,7] With that information, occupational therapists were then able to plan programs more specifically, not only for the tuberculous patient, but also for patients with cardiac problems, chronic obstructive pulmonary disease, or for anyone requiring habit training to match a reduced vital capacity or energy level. And still today, application of this more precise knowledge of energy expenditure for activities makes it possible to structure programs more exactly, not only for the patient with a given cardiac classification but for any person with a problem of low energy.[5,6]

During the 1940's and 1950's many therapists were working with patients with poliomyelitis who required individual treatment programs because of diverse patterns of residual paralysis. One caveat for therapists then was not to over-fatigue any muscle. Accordingly, body alignment was maintained to eliminate gravity so that weakened muscles could perform at least some elementary activity.[8] Work with polio patients resulted in occupational therapists developing many kinds of adapted equipment and methods to help these patients and others achieve maximum independence despite minimal residual strength.[9,10,11] This technology and methods for teaching activities of daily living have become so standard within the profession that they are commonplace in textbooks.[12,13,14,15]

Some professionals criticized occupational therapists for demanding too much effort from patients to achieve small gains in functional ability, even when patients obviously were never going to return to their former motor capacities.[16] While not disagreeing, Reilly described occupational therapists as "having blind devotion to the belief that every patient has a right to physical independence."[17,p202] Most occupational therapists subscribed to the work ethic, so common among people of the United States, and assumed that patients whom they treated shared that work ethic and to a large extent that was true.

As a result, for the goal of maximum function within the limits of whatever disability, therapists began in the 1950's and 1960's to devise equipment and methods that could make almost any task less strenuous to perform, or to make it possible to perform in spite of many physical limitations. This was the time that dressing routines using one extremity, or with loss of range of motion, or with involuntary movement, were developed and codified.[9,10] These practices were developed to help patients accomplished self-care activities that therapists felt were so important for the patient to perform independently.

General technological advances have made many daily living and work activities easier for everyone. Changes in fabrics and a more casual form of dress have made clothing easier to put on and take off and to care for. New design and technology in home appliances have certainly made care of one's home less difficult. And improvement in food technology, including ways of preparing food, means that each meal does not have to be prepared from scratch. All these changes have significantly reduced the amounts of effort now needed to perform chores that used to require more time and energy. And most recently, the development of personal computers opens many opportunities for independence and increased efficiency in communication, work and environmental controls for everyone, but especially for the energy deficient patient.[18]

However, although many of these advances are the accepted norm for the middle income family, where using technologics to conserve energy may be commonplace, they may not be accessible for those in large, low income families. Then, traditional methods for doing activities may still need to be planned.

WHAT IS ENERGY?

The concept of low energy related to patient abilities is best described and understood by examining the literature on the physiology of energy and work.[19] Physiologically energy is described as biological and is divided into the elements of internal work and external work. *Internal work* relates to the resting metabolic rate or the energy consumed for maintenance of normal body functions. It is estimated to comprise about sixty percent of one's total expenditure of energy and goes on even while the body is at rest.[20] There is additional internal energy used by the thermic effect of food and the production of extra heat for a period after eating. This 'adaptive thermogenesis', the adaptive changes in that rate due to temperature, eating, emotional stress and environmental conditions, adds to the resting metabolic rate. Although adaptive thermogenesis may account for no more than ten to fifteen percent change in the resting metabolic rate, this variability may be an important consideration for therapists as they assess energy balance within diverse environmental conditions. For example, most of the energy produced by the body as a result of eating is taken up with body maintenance to achieve physiological homeostasis.[20]

External work, or movement—the contraction of skeletal muscles for any activity—is the most variable amount of 'work' and daily demands vary in that energy expenditure depends on the intensity and duration of a particular activity. However, this residual percentage of total energy available may be all an energy deficient patient has for all ADL's.[20] Physiologists relate energy output to food intake. This equation balances intake with human functions. However, as occupational therapists know, there is difference between the *basic need* activities and the *discretionary* activities people engage in outside of 'working' time. With energy, perhaps more than with nutrients, both physiological and socio-psychological elements of human behavior must be considered. Discussion of energy therefore should always involve concepts from both the biological and social sciences. Thereby one focuses on the importance of basic needs relative to survival, versus discretionary uses of energy for higher level needs and self-actualization.[21]

WORK: WHAT WE KNOW AND HOW WE APPLY IT

Work, the most variable continuum of energy use, has been studied extensively in industry to improve work efficiency, reduce fatigue and increase safety.[22] However, because the energy expenditure measures reported resulted from observations in specific working conditions and environments, those measures are of little value in estimating energy demands under other conditions. Interpretations of 'total energy expenditures for a day' have limitations.[23] Studies also show that an individual's energy balance varies greatly from week to week, and even day to day within weeks. Energy is used with variable efficiency as the body attempts to maintain homeostasis. Little is known of how energy utilization for work may be varied, and total requirements for maintaining body function, including temperature, are still unknown. The body regulates energy balance by changing the efficiency of energy utilization. Energy requirements of humans and their efficiency in using it varies greatly because of intra-individual variation.[24]

It is known that daily levels of 'usual activity' have positive effects on physical work capacity. However, it is necessary to take into consideration both the kind of work and its duration, and the other factors related to activity habits and motor performance, to estimate anyone's daily potential for activity. These other factors include age, sex, size, body composition as well as health and nutritional status and many other socio-cultural circumstances.[25,26]

Reducing one's activity level is a way of achieving energy balance. This is an adaptive mechanism that imposes restrictions that may be costly to the individual's adjustment to the ecological and cultural context in which he lives. There is little information on how the behavioral nature of activities may be affected by this adaptive mechanism.[27] It may be that energy deficient people find more efficient ways of doing set tasks. Since physical activity (external work) accounts for about a third of daily energy expenditure, any savings in energy costs for activities must be planned by taking into consideration overall energy requirments.[28]

OCCUPATIONAL THERAPY ALTERS THE ILLUSIVE FACTOR

Physical Means

Energy conservation measures are well described in occupational therapy textbooks.[12,13,14,15] They relate to the organization of activities, simplified means to accomplish a task, planning, alternating heavy and light tasks—all techniques well known to occupational therapists. The energy deficient patient, for whatever reason, may have diminished *strength* which makes even small tasks difficult.

Yet, many strength building techniques require large sustained outputs of muscular effort or energy as, for example, the DeLorme techniques of progressive resistive exercise which require the exerciser to perform from 10 to 50 muscle contractions against maximum resistance for a given bout.[29] Another exercise technique may be considered as more feasible for the energy deficient patient in an effort to build strength to make functional activities easier. That technique is BRIME, *BR*ief, *I*sometric, *M*aximal *E*xercise, in which contractions of only five to six seconds duration are used with a 20 second interval between contractions. Although prolonged isometric exercise is contraindicated for patients with cardiovascular problems, the BRIME are short, and studies of their use have not shown increases in blood pressure during the exercise.[30] Use of this exercise technique could be considered by occupational therapists for the energy deficient patient who could profit by greater strength to accomplish basic need activities.

In addition to using the suggestions for strength building and the information available on energy conservation techniques, occupational therapists may also teach energy deficient patients new ways to do some ADL's by using central nervous system reflexes that coordinate large groups of muscles. Specific techniques are based on known qualities associated with reflexes. For example, reflexes tend to bias the musculature in favor of movement in the direction of gaze. The tonic labyrinthine reflexes, body on head, tonic neck reflex, and body on body righting are such. It is suggested that the nervous system produces an economy of movement and therefore the reflexes yield coordinative movement rather than having to plan a movement of individual muscle contractions. Although the resulting movements are based on reflexes they have a more volitional appearance.[31]

Occupational therapists are accustomed to using reflex evaluation in their work with children. Occupational therapists assess the extent of the influence of reflexes on movement and treat in ways to inhibit reflexes that lock a child into obligatory movement patterns. This information on early human development can also be applied to efforts at developing economy of movement for an older person or for the energy deficient patient. For example, when moving in bed, a person can be taught to look in the direction of movement, turning his head to that side; the shoulders and hips will follow easily, an example of the neck righting reaction acting on the body.[32] Or, for sitting up from supine in bed, while lying on one's side with the hips and knees slightly flexed, it is relatively easy to place the legs over the edge of the bed, capitalizing on the influence of gravity. Then the person pushes with the arms to assume the final erect position. This method is easier than coming to a sitting position abruptly without arm support, from supine. It is the method often suggested for people having back pain and the method actually is applicable to achieving the upright position more easily for any of us.[33]

Standing up from a chair can be made easier for an energy deficient patient by arranging a chair with elongated legs or a raised seat. More energy is consumed in standing up from a chair whose height equals just the length of the foreleg, that is, from the heel to the tibial plateau, than when the chair seat is raised to be 1-1/5 the height of the foreleg. Even less energy is required when the chair height is 1-1/2 times the length of the foreleg.[34] Standing up from a chair without pushing up with the arms can become a strengthening exercise if the height of the seat is gradually reduced over time.[32,35] Use of flexion and extension patterns can also facilitate standing up from a chair. The person is instructed to scoot forward to the edge of the chair, place feet about 12 inches apart for a good base, lean forward, bending at the hips and neck. This puts a slight stretch on the back extensors. Then the patient is instructed to look up as he stands up; this promotes an extensor pattern to facilitate coming to the upright position.[35]

Energy is related to motor output or contraction of skeletal muscles. The improvement of motor ability for the energy deficient patient may also be helped by teaching motor learning through still other facilitation and inhibition techniques. One such group of techniques particularly applicable to adult functional activities is Proprioceptive Neuromuscular Facilitation (PNF). Techniques for facilitating the patient toward more efficient motor function are outlined by Voss, Ionta and Myers.[36] A principle of PNF uses a diagonal pattern of motion to elicit the stretch reflex. It is possible to teach activities of daily living through the use of these diagonal patterns of movement. If, as suggested by Easton,[31] use of reflexes promotes an economy of movement, and diagonal patterns facilitate the use of reflexes, then a combination of the two methods should provide the energy deficient patient with one more means for more efficient use of energy expended in daily activities.

PSYCHO-SOCIAL CONSIDERATIONS

Americans are independent and work oriented.[37,38] For those who must reduce their amount of daily activity because of a medical problem, a process of restructuring attitudes is as needed as physical means for generating alternate choices within the realm of the patient's ability. The value system of work and independence that prevails in American culture may make it difficult for those with chronic debilitating diseases to relinquish to others some of their independence for activities of daily living or to give up their own ways of performing activities. For example, a lady with a Gower's Sign (from muscular dystrophy) insisted on scrubbing her floors on hands and knees rather than using any kind of mop. Klavins and Sanchez[39,40] each point out that occupational therapists need to realize that work values are not universal and they suggest that approaches to patients should fit the patient's values. Thus they would better help individuals to conform to some patterns of behavior and performance acceptable within patients' life styles and to personal support systems available.[41,42]

Most adults are creatures of habit and perform tasks much the way they learned to do them as children, or while observing parents and relatives trying to accomplish a given activity. Others who find themselves devastated with a medical problem that limits energy and function may not have considered alternate methods of doing things they cannot now do, and may be very pleased to have a therapist instruct them in different ways of performing them.

With improvements in knowledge, skills and techniques in the practice of medicine and surgery, many people now are alive but have little or significantly diminished energy available to perform the work they want to do every day. They are the patients with disabling heart attacks, not the ones who can exercise on a treadmill to monitor their recovery, but those who are precarious and may not be permitted to do any physical activity; the individual with arthritis who may have systemic anemia that makes activity difficult; those with lung diseases who are unable to achieve enough vital capacity to support activity in the usual way. Others with residual weakness from spinal cord injury, cerebral vascular accident, and other disabling conditions find that ordinary activities are most difficult and exertion may make them too tired to think or to devote time to more creative activities. Should a therapeutic goal with these patients be directed toward their becoming more independent in activities of daily living? Inevitably patients will choose to engage in things they consider important, but an occupational therapist can make those choices less stringent by showing patients alternatives.

The Independent Living Movement (ILM) is one outcome of

unmet needs of disabled people. The disabled themselves are interested in solving their own problems in ways they choose and implement. The proponents of the ILM suggest that society should support the disabled person so that he can live the life style that gives him the greatest satisfaction. That means the disabled choose what they do with their available energy. Writers for the ILM ask society, for example, to compare the relative merits of a disabled person who is dressed by an attendant and then goes to work, versus that person using two hours to dress independently and then being too tired to go to work and thus remaining at home.[43]

CONCLUSION

Although occupational therapists have traditionally focused on helping patients achieve maximum physical and mental function through participation in selected activities, there has always been the patient who could do very little 'work' because of paralysis or other characteristics of a disability or illness. Therapists have always found methods to assist most patients to achieve maximum function by inventing different ways to plan or solve problems within current capacities. Although many of the resulting devices and techniques for engaging patients have become standard for practice in the profession, the therapist is always challenged by still another group of patients who survive but barely 'live' due to advanced technologies in medical care. It is then usualy left to others to help make the life saved worth living. Occupational therapists, by teaching patients skills and techniques to achieve some measure of independence and satisfaction, play a large role in helping persons find that worth.

REFERENCES

1. Pollitt E, Amante P, Editors: Energy Intake and Activity. NY: Alan R. Liss, Inc., 1984

2. Wade BD: Occupational Therapy for Patients with Mental Disease, p 81-139 in Principles of Occupational Therapy edited by HS Willard, CS Spackman. Philadelphia: JB Lippincott Co., 1947

3. Hudson H: Occupational Therapy for the Tuberculous, p 301-316 in Principles of Occupational Therapy edited by HS Willard, CS Spackman. Philadelphia: JB Lippincott Co., 1947

4. Gordon EE, Haas A: Energy cost during various physical activites in convalescing tuberculosis patients. *AM Rev Tuberculosis* 71:724-728, 1955

5. Hendrickson D, et al.: Physiological approach to the regulation of activity in the cardiac convalescent. *Am J Occup Ther* 14:292-296, 1960

6. Kottke F: Study of cardiac output during rehabilitation activities. *Arch Phys Med* 38:79, 1957

7. Passmore R, Durnin JVGA: Human energy expenditure. *Physiol Rev* 35:801-840, 1955

8. Dargan FP: Occupational therapy for the poliomyelitic. *Am J Occup Ther* 9: 272-27, 1955

9. Emmett R: Adaptation of homemaking skills for the hemiplegic woman. *Am J Occup Ther* 11:283-287, 290, 1957

10. Brett G: Dressing techniques for the severely involved hemiplegic patient. *Am J Occup Ther* 14:262-264, 1960

11. Klinger JL: Activities of daily living: Some comments on recent developments. *Am J Occup Ther* 19:295-299, 1965

12. Hopkins HL, Smith HD: Willard and Spackman's Occupational Therapy, 6th edition. Philadelphia: JB Lippincott, 1983

13. Lewis CB: Aging: The Health Care Challenge. Philadelphia: FA Davis Co., 1985

14. Pedretti LW: Occupational Therapy, Practice Skills for Physical Dysfunction. St. Louis: CV Mosby Co., 1981

15. Trombly CA: Occupational Therapy for Physical Dysfunction, 2nd edition. Baltimore: Williams & Wilkins, 1983

16. Myerson L: Some observations on the psychological roles of the occupational therapist. *Am J Occup Ther* 11:131-134

17. Reilly MA: Letter to the Editor. *Am J Occup Ther* 11:202-203, 1957

18. McWilliams P: Personal Computers and the Disabled. New York: Quantum Press/Doubleday, 1984

19. Astrand PO, Rodahl K: Textbook of Work Physiology, Physiological Bases of Exercise, 2nd edition. New York: McGraw Hill Book Co., 1977

20. Horton ES: Appropriate Methodology for Assessing Physical Activity Under Laboratory Conditions in Studies of Energy Balance in Adults. In Energy Intake and Activity, E Pollitt and P Amante, Editors. New York: Alan R. Liss, Inc., 1984

21. Beaton GH: Adaptation to and Accommodation of Long Term Low Energy Intake: A Commentary on the Conference on Energy Intake and Activity. In Energy Intake and Activity, E Pollitt, P Amante, Editors. New York: Alan R. Liss, Inc. 1984

22. Brun T: Physiological Measurement of Activity Among Adults Under Free Living Conditions. In Energy Intake and Activity, E Pollitt, P Amante, Editors. New York: Alan R. Liss, Inc., 1984

23. Durnin JVGA: Some Problems in Assessing the Role of Physical Activity in the Maintenance of Energy Balance. In Energy Intake and Activity, E Pollitt and P Amante, Editors. New York: Alan R. Liss, Inc., 1984

24. Margen S: Auto-Regulator Processes and Energy Balance In Energy Intake and Activity, E Pollitt and P Amante, Editors. New York: Alan R. Liss, Inc., 1984

25. Malina RM: Physical Activity and Motor Development/Performance in Populations Nutritionally at Risk. In Energy Intake and Activity, E Pollitt and P Amante, Editors. New York: Alan R. Liss, Inc., 1984

26. Spurr GB: Nutritional Status and Physical Work Capacity in Relation to Agricultural Productivity. In Energy Intake and Activity, E Pollitt, P Amante, Editors. New York: Alan R. Liss, Inc., 1984

27. Scrimshaw NS, Pollitt E: Preface. Energy Intake and Activity, E Pollitt, P. Amante, Editors. New York: Alan R. Liss, Inc., 1984

28. Prentice AM: Adaptations to Long-Term Low Energy Intake. In Energy Intake and Activity, E Pollitt, P Amante, Editors. New York: Alan R. Liss, Inc., 1984

29. Schram DA: Resistance Exercise, p 191-200 in Therapeutic Exercise, 3rd Edition. JV Basmajian, Editor. Baltimore: Williams & Wilkins, 1978

30. Liberson WT: Brief Isometric Exercises, p 201-209 in Therapeutic Exercise, 3rd Edition. JV Basmajian, Editor. Baltimore: Williams & Wilkins, 1978

31. Easton TA: On the normal use of reflexes. *Am Sci* 60:591-599, 1972

32. Barnes MR, Crutchfield CA, Heriza CB: The Neurophysiological Basis of Patient Treatment, Volume II, Reflexes in Motor Development. Morgantown, WVA: Stokesville Publishing Co., 1978

33. Hirschberg GG, Lewis L, Vaughn P: Rehabilitation: A Manual for the Care of the Disabled and Elderly, 2nd edition. Philadelphia: JB Lippincott, 1976

34. Hirschberg GG, et al.: Energy cost of stand-up exercises in normal and hemiplegic subjects. *Am J Phys Med* 42-143-145, 1964

35. Sine RD, et al.: Basic Rehabilitation Techniques. Germantown, MD: Aspen Systems Corp., 1977

36. Voss DE, Ionta MK, Myers BJ: Proprioceptive Neuromuscular Facilitation: Patterns and Techniques, 3rd edition. New York: Harper and Row, 1985

37. Kluckhohn F, Strodtbeck FL: Variations in Value Orientations. Evanston IL: Row, Peterson and Co., 1962

38. Lerner M: America As a Civilization. New York: Simon & Schuster, 1957

39. Klavins R: The relevance of work-play theory to human adaptation: Work play behavior: Cultural influences. *Am J Occup Ther* 26:176-178, 1972

40. Sanchez V: Relevance of cultural values for occupational therapy programs. *Am J Occup Ther* 18:1-5, 1964

41. Barris R, Kielhofner G: Early and Middle Adulthood, p 112-122 in A Model of Human Occupation, Theory and Application. Edited by G. Kielhofner. Baltimore: Williams & Wilkins, 1985

42. Rogers JC, Snow TL: Later Adulthood, p 123-133 in A Model of Human Occupation, Theory and Application. Edited by G. Kielhofner. Baltimore: Williams & Wilkins, 1985

43. DeJong G: Independent living: From social movement to analytic paradigm. *Arch Phys Med Rehabil* 60:435-445, 1979

Designing Environments
for the Elderly

Mary Grace Washburn, MHA, OTR, FAOTA

ABSTRACT. Planning living environments for the elderly is a challenge due to the variety of characteristics and the changing health status of this special population. An occupational therapist's knowledge and understanding of the aging process, as well as the profession's philosophy of maximizing health through active living can contribute to the design of retirement centers. The concepts and basic principles involved in such collaborative planning are discussed. This paper concludes with an invocation for more occupational therapists to seek opportunities to be involved in facility planning for the elderly.

Designing living environments for the elderly is challenging because of the multiplicity of changes that occur in a person's experience of the aging process. One of the prevalent changes that affects life style patterns in aging persons is decreasing energy. This potential change, as well as other factors, must be considered if one is to design environments for the elderly. Specially designed environments facilitate maximum independent functioning regardless of the stage of the aging process or dysfunction due to age or disability.

Mary Grace Washburn is a healthcare consultant who assists hospitals and developers in the development of alternative living and programs for the elderly. Her experience also includes working with an architectural firm which designed healthcare facilities. As an occupational therapist, Ms. Washburn worked with the elderly in both hospitals and long term care facilities.

This article appears jointly in *Occupational Therapy for the Energy Deficient Patient* (The Haworth Press, 1986) and *Occupational Therapy in Health Care,* Volume 3, Number 1 (Spring 1986).

17

In the recent past, design of buildings for the elderly, such as nursing homes, has been motivated by demand for efficiency by those caring for the residents. In these dehumanizing environments dependency is promoted and residents slowly deteriorate. Further, such 'efficient' settings and other environments for the elderly similiarly designed, have served to 'disconnect' the elderly from living. In addition, an approach such as in the 'Sun City' type of community design (communities which are remote from urban resources) assumes that retired persons want to be isolated from the mainstream and will also remain independent and active as they age. Today, the issues of such communities center on how to care for those who have dysfunction and are now slightly dependent. In addition, it is found that many residents are feeling a social void without the interaction with younger people. Obviously not all the needs of older persons were considered in planning these environments.

With a sharp increase in the number of elderly persons, an enlightened attention toward designing functional living arrangements for the elderly is occurring. Some developers, however, are still perpetuating the generic designs of the past or are being swept into the latest trends in general architectural design as suitable for the elderly. Others, fortunately, are striving to create environments which reflect both understanding of the needs of and a caring attitude for the older person.[3] These environments are created to promote health, to facilitate continuing functional abilities, to provide or have available specific assistance as persons require it, and to recognize and accommodate preferences for different life styles.

An occupational therapist's philosophy and understanding of the healthy aging process can be important contributions to the development and the concept of environments for the elderly. Occupational therapists have the ability to visualize a person performing physical and social tasks in his total environment. Effective design is accomplished when there is a close relationship between physical design, behavior and purpose.[4] This special expertise can be offered to developers who do not possess the special insights about the elderly. With this approach, developers can design a living environment which will accommodate persons of all stages of aging, with varying abilities and interests.

The following discussion presents both some of the basic concepts and the criteria for designing environments for the aged, based on occupational therapy philosophies.

THE CONCEPTS

The concepts for specially designed environments for the elderly must be based on a *health* care philosophy. It, therefore, must recognize 'the whole person', the individuality of people and the varying process and effects of aging. Environments created must facilitate health, not simply take care of sickness. Healthy environments foster and encourage independence, involvement, socialization, mental stimulation and psychological well-being. Occupational therapists are committed to promoting these environments in which the quality of life is valued.[5]

Considering the effects of aging and factors related to specific dysfunctions, one must design elderly environments to accommodate a continuum of care. The continuum must offer various levels of care both for those who are active and independent as well as for those who have varying degrees and kinds of dependency. These 'levels of living and care' are represented usually by retirement apartments or cottages for those who are independent, by special residential and personal care arrangments for those who require minimal assistance for mental functioning or supervision for daily activities, and by nursing services for those who require constant care or supervision. Continuing care retirement and life care communities offer these levels of living and care—a continuum of care. This means that when persons move into communities they can remain for their lifetime even though their functional status may change due to either the aging process or subsequent disability.

The continuum of care environment facilitates maximum independence through allowing persons to maintain their usual routines, participate in purposeful activities and have opportunities for socialization. The environment accommodates to individual needs. Supportive care, when provided is individual and is integrated into a living environment rather than being provided in a traditional institutional atmosphere. Nursing care when needed is given in still familiar settings close to friends and one's most recent living environment.

Older adults who wish to remain healthy and live out their lives with dignity strive to find such an environment for living which will enhance and satisfy healthy aging. There are a number of fundamental principles to guide the successful development of environments for the elderly. Many reflect basic occupational therapy philosophies for optimum adaptation. These will now be discussed.

CRITERIA FOR DESIGNING ENVIRONMENTS FOR THE ELDERLY

I. Facilitate Functional Abilities to Allow Maximum Independence

M. Powell Lawton, a well-known researcher in environmental designs for the elderly, created the ecological model for the design of health care environments. He states that the purpose of his ecological model is the match between supportiveness of the setting and a person's ability to cope. A person's competency (his physical, mental and emotional abilities) must match the 'environmental press'. Environmental press is the degree of difficulty of living demanded from or associated with a health care environment. Low environmental press is the most 'supportive', such as that found in a nursing home. Therefore, a person with a low level of competency will be most comfortable in a setting with low environmental press. If a person's environment is mismatched with his needs, he will not only be uncomfortable but will have difficulty managing as well.[6]

Just as one with dysfunction adjusts if provided the appropriate equipment or assistance with activities of daily living, so must he live in an environment with the appropriate amount of support.

A person's interaction with the environment defines his level of dysfunction or function. In order to provide the appropriate amount of environmental support to each individual, there must be some flexibility in the planning of environments. But from a practical point of view, units within a retirement center cannot be individually designed; they may, however, provide the opportunity for varied arrangements and modifications which allow residents to effectively accomplish daily activities. Supportive measures such as handrails in bathrooms may not be necessary for all residents but should, nevertheless, be planned for and installed in all units. Thus, such features would be placed unobtrusively and be functional aids incorporated as design features rather than 'add-ons'. Having too many aids may signal a feeling of being handicapped to some residents. therefore, careful initial design based on the functional expectations of older people can provide the right match of setting for optimum and continuing independence.

II. Compensate for Aging Factors Such as Diminishing Energy, Lowered Sensory and Perceptual Abilities and Problems in Orientation

It is well documented that the aging process introduces changes in physical, sensory and perceptual abilities.[7,8,9] With some persons the changes are slight; with others the changes may significantly interfere with daily functioning. In designing environments, therefore, various structural features, conditions, and products can be incorporated to help anticipate and compensate for such changes and limitations. For example, distances between rooms, acessibility to common areas, activities, exits and walkways must be evaluated so that persons with limited energy or difficulty walking can manage. Further, for those in apartments or cottages, the amount of reaching, standing, bending and carrying to perform household and food preparation activities is important in kitchen and storage designs.

Commonly, the eyesight of the elderly decreases, making it difficult in certain lighting to respond or adapt readily to environmental/structural changes.[10] A consistent intensity of light with no dim light within the public spaces and living quarters will ease the strain on the eyesight of the elderly.

Due to sensory deficits and disease conditions, the elderly may experience perceptual difficulties. Since distinguishing subtle differences in color, identifying obstacles in a path or operating complicated locks may be problematic, environments should be planned to anticipate such difficulties. Providing for successful function must take precedence over 'style and artistry'.

Some elderly persons have difficulty with orientation to time and space. Therefore it is helpful if the living environments can be arranged to have similarities to recent living accommodations. For example, doors and windows might operate similarly to those most commonly used in residential homes.[11] Arrangement of furniture and appliances in familiar places is also a technique which aids in maintaining orientation.

III. Allow for Individual Choices

Allowing an individual some choices to personalize his own living space helps to maintain his self-esteem, confidence and decision making abilities. Each person relocating to senior housing will have had his own unique lifestyle and may prefer variations in space use. For example, one may prefer to have a dining room rather than a kitchen eating area. Moveable partitions or screens can facilitate such choices in space use.

IV. Create a Balance Between Privacy and Socialization

The way a facility is designed has significant impact on both privacy and opportunities for socialization. Designing social areas which branch off of the primary path encourages social encounters but does not force socialization.[12] Circulation paths and benches on the exterior grounds can be laid out to bring about friendly meetings. Lounges near areas used routinely such as the laundry room provide natural gathering places. Some persons whose activities are limited enjoy being able to watch others in activities; a balcony above the activity area can make this sharing possible. With open public spaces, informal conversational and private groupings can be created simply through the arrangement of furniture and tables. At the same time, design of individual space must allow for privacy, both for the resident and visiting guests. Of older residents of institutional settings, visiting is the most satisfying activity.[13]

V. Encourage Active Participation

Many rooms or areas designated for activities in facilities for the elderly are vacant because they do not invite purposeful activity and interpersonal exchange. Activity areas which do encourage involvement of residents might include a small store, an ice cream parlor, garden, an active library, small offices for persons who can offer services (such as legal advice or party arrangements), a flower shop, club areas (literary, camera, philately, card games) or study group areas. Other avenues for activity occur when general kitchen/dining areas are designed to allow residents to assist with meal preparation, table setting, clean-up, and beverage serving.

Day care centers can be connected to an elderly living environment and thereby provide opportunities for residents to interact with children. In addition, if space is available for individual or group flower and vegetable gardens, this offers other avenues not only for shared participation and personal enrichment but exercise as well. These types of activities provide residents an opportunity to demonstrate skills, to give to others, and to build self-esteem. An integral part of the 'future oriented' design will be areas for *work,* not busy work.[14]

VI. Provide Safety and Security

Safety and security are two important factors that guide persons as they select special environments for living. Thus provisions must be planned to assure these aspects of facility operation. In most facilities, regardless of location or design, to assure security it is essential to monitor those who enter the grounds and/or the facility. For the latter a buzzer system at the front entry is most commonly used; otherwise security gates or actual guards are used. The outdoor areas may need to be enclosed or access monitored to prevent mildly confused residents from wandering away. This protective environment alleviates the fear of crime and is an advantage much sought as compared to living within the community.[15]

Safety is accomplished by careful attention to design of all building elements: stair and curb heights, flooring materials and coverings, lighting, door handles, as well as furniture and appliance size and design to fit persons who may be smaller in size and with less strength and balance.

An emergency button and intercom system is commonly installed within each resident's unit to aid in quick response by the staff in case of emergencies. Parking areas for residents' cars must also provide for both safety and security. Sophisticated fire alarm systems and smoke detectors are essential as well as carefully planned exits and passageways to accommodate exit for persons who use aids for walking and wheelchairs. Because of both physical and sensory limitations of residents such arrangements must be clearly identified and rehearsed.

VII. Integration With the Community

When designing an environment for the elderly, consideration should be given to ways in which the residents can relate to the surrounding community. Access to public transportation, churches, shopping areas, beauty parlor and barber shop, bank, post office, and a park should be considered.[15]

Integration with the community can be accomplished by being located close to an adjoining day care center, a sports field, a park or a community center where others from the community gather. Careful consideration to the location of elderly living can encourage and enhance continual participation in community activities and offer opportunity for a community support network for the residents.

CONCLUSION

Designing living environments for the elderly requires a comprehensive approach that considers all aspects of residents' characteristics and functional abilities both current and future. It entails consideration not just of the physcial features of a building, admittedly important, but more important, an assessment of how the elder person will manage, physically, socially and psychologically within the environment to continue a healthy, active life. With careful thought to the criteria described and their incorporation into design plans, a facility can promote health and facilitate active and safe functioning for residents. The occupational therapist's knowledge and philosophies can make a significant difference in the effectiveness of the resulting environment for the elderly. It is important for occupational therapists to be involved in the architectural design as well as in the planning of programs and services for the special environments for the elderly. Given the demographics of tomorrow, there is great opportunity for this kind of participation by occupational therapists who market their skills in this direction.

REFERENCES

1. Bush, R: "The age of aging." *Prog Archit* 8: p. 59-63, 1981
2. Morton, D: "Congregate living." *Prog Archit* 8: p. 64-68, 1981
3. Lindhe, R: "Environments for the elderly: future oriented design for living?" *J Archit Educ,* Vol. 27, No. 1,2, p. 7-10, 55-56, 1974
4. Dunning, H; "Environmental occupational therapy." *Am J Occ Ther* 26: p. 262-97
5. . . . . Official position paper: "Occupational therapy's role in independent or alternative living situations." *Am J Occ Ther* 35: p. 812-13, 1981
6. Byerts, T, Regnier, V: "Applying research to the plan and design of housing for the elderly." Housing for a Mature Population. Washington: Urban Land Institution, p. 2526, 1983
7. Lewis, S: "The Mature Years: A geriatric occupational therapy text." Chas. B. Slack, NJ, 1979
8. Green, I, Fedewa, B, Johnston, C, Jackson, W, Deardorff, H: Housing for the Elderly: The Development and Design Process. Van Nostrand Rheinhold, Co., 1975
9. Jordan, J: "Recognizing and designing for the special needs of the elderly." *AIA J* 66: p. 50-55, 1977

10. Editor: "Aging eyes demand special design." *Indus Design* 29: p. 12, 1982
11. Stephens, S: "Hidden barriers." *Prog Archit* 4: p. 94-97, 1978
12. Howell, S: Designing for the Elderly. MIT, MA, 1980
13. Tickle, L, Yerxa, E: "Need satisfaction of older persons living in the community and institutions, part II—role of activity." *Am J Occ Ther* 35: p. 650-655, 1981
14. Ibid. 3
15. Tickle, L, Yerxa, E: "Need satisfaction of older persons living in the community and in institutions, part I—the environment." *Am J Occ Ther* 35: p. 645-649, 1981
16. Ibid. 8

Outcomes of a Problem-Solving Approach to Independence in Children With Multiple Limb Deficiencies: A Case Study of Adaptation to the Demands of Adulthood

Susan D. Clarke, MA, OTR

ABSTRACT. Occupational therapists can play a unique role in helping children with disabilities develop a positive history of mastery of skills and habits necessary for continued movement along the developmental continuum throughout the life cycle. An independent problem-solving approach to treatment is suggested as a method of facilitating development of skills and habits which will continue to support independence. A case history of a 27-year-old woman who as a child participated in a program using this approach illustrates her use of independent problem-solving to master competent performance of adult roles.

Coping with a disability which compromises energy levels is a life-long process for persons who have a congenital disability or are disabled early in childhood. As developmental tasks change with age, so do demands on limited energy resources. Groundwork for developing patterns of adaptation to best use existing physical and emotional energy potential must begin early in the treatment of these children. The occupational therapist is in a key position to assist the

Susan D. Clarke is a clinical therapist, educator, and researcher at the Child Amputee Prosthetics Project at UCLA. She is a graduate of the University of New Hampshire and the Graduate School of the University of Southern California.

This article appears jointly in *Occupational Therapy for the Energy Deficient Patient* (The Haworth Press, 1986) and *Occupational Therapy in Health Care*, Volume 3, Number 1 (Spring 1986).

27

child in developing the necessary skills, habits, and decision-making abilities to maximize potential use of adaptation for mastering changing developmental demands throughout the life cycle.

In adult rehabilitation there is a tendency to focus on specific solutions to specific problems as roles and habits are well established and reasonably stable. A history of functional adaptation already exists in individuals who become disabled later in life. This serves as a reservoir of skills and habits that can be used and modified to meet the changing needs imposed by disability.[1] In working with children, the therapist is intimately involved in creating this history of skills and habits upon which future adaptation will depend. It is especially important because demands for acquisition of new skills, habits and roles are constant as the child progresses through the developmental continuum. In order to develop a sense of efficacy and competence in adulthood, children with disabilities must develop a history of skills and habits which will allow them to problem-solve and make decisions about the demands placed on them by the roles of adulthood. Only then will they be able to take control of their lives and become independent.

Different disabilities place different demands on a child in terms of the degree of adaptation they must make in order to become independent. Children with multiple limb deficiencies must first master prostheses, if they are appropriate, and then integrate use of them into their activities of daily living. Although their disability is stable, it continues to compromise energy levels to an increasingly greater extent with age as they increase in size and body weight and their roles demand greater independence and performance of more complex and time consuming tasks.

In order to analyze the effectiveness of a treatment program designed for persons with developmental disabilities such as multiple limb deficiencies, it is necessary to select a theory and rationale for treatment which encompasses the entire life cycle. A system must also be developed to analyze both short and long-term effects of treatment. In this instance long term means years and, at best, is a sampling of results at intervals throughout the life cycle.[2] Few rehabilitation settings currently provide opportunities for such long-term follow-up. The Child Amputee Prosthetics Project (CAPP) at the University of California at Los Angeles is able to conduct such studies for a number of reasons. The staff has developed a unique expertise in care of children and young adults with limb deficiencies because of the selectivity of the caseload, the funding sources available for care as well as research, and the continuity of staff throughout its history. This history not only allows the staff to offer services not available elsewhere in the community, but also encourages the patients to maintain a liaison with the clinic over time.

THEORETICAL APPROACH TO TREATMENT

This article is based on the research and experience of the staff at CAPP. The theoretical basis for treatment planning for the past 30 years has been a normal growth and development model.[3] The method of treatment has been based on an independent problem-solving approach to mastery of new tasks.[4]

The rationale for selecting this combination of theory and method was based on the assumption that human growth and development requires a constantly changing repertoire of skills and habits to progress normally. Therefore, it was not enough to train children to perform specific tasks such as learning to operate a prosthesis or mastery of developmental milestones, they must also be assisted in acquiring the ability to apply and modify current skills to meet the changing demands of normal developmental progress without assistance when at all possible. Only this ability would lead to the spontaneous and effective inclusion of the prosthesis in everyday activities throughout the life cycle.

Because of CAPP's long history, beginning in the early 1950s, the knowledge base for this methodological approach to treatment has grown with time. The introduction of Piaget's theories on cognitive development has greatly enhanced the levels to which developmental theory can be incorporated into treatment planning. He has done much to explain the role of independent problem-solving in normal development beginning with his descriptions of accommodation and assimilation.[5]

The development of a model of human occupation as defined by Kielhofner and Burke has also provided a framework which can be used to examine the treatment process in its totality. According to this model, ''all human occupation arises out of an innate spontaneous tendency of the human system—the urge to explore and master the environment.''[6] This model also incorporates the importance of skills ''flexibly organised and interrelated component actions that lead to the accomplishment of a purpose of goal under variable environmental conditions''[6] and habits (certain actions repeated by an individual which become routine) to the development of competent behaviors throughout the life cycle.[6]

Recent research in learning theory on contextual interference effect (the interference that results from practicing a task within the context of a practice session) has also added to the rationale behind a problem-solving approach to mastery of new tasks. It has shown that high contextual interference (more variety in the presentation and types of practice situations) leads to better long term skill acquisition.[7]

The independent problem-solving approach to mastery of new tasks used at CAPP to assist children in developing prosthetic skills, habits of prosthetic use, and mastery of activities of daily living, is best operationally defined by describing the process. The therapist selects a developmentally appropriate task and presents it to the child with a demonstration or description of the expected end result. The child is asked to complete the task without assistance. Assistance is given only when the child is unable to complete the task. He or she is then given suggestions or demonstrations of how the task might be completed. If the task is completed in a less than optimum manner, the child is rewarded for his success and encouraged to improve his or her performance. Direct instruction on right or wrong ways to master a task are avoided. Mastery of different ways to accomplish the same task is encouraged. All appropriate behaviors are rewarded as they occur. In this manner the child learns the important task of independent problem-solving while mastering appropriate developmental skills.

The following example illustrates the application of this approach to the mastery of new tasks. A 5-year-old child with bilateral above-elbow prostheses is presented with the task of placing a spoon in her dominant hook. She has had previous experience with placement of long objects, such as drum sticks and paint brushes, which require prepositioning of the hook in the wrist unit. The child is seated with a spoon and plate on the table in front of her and is asked to pick up the spoon and see if she can get it to her mouth. She can grab it by the raised end of the bowl, but not the handle.

> *Therapist*: How can you get a hold of the handle?
> *Child*: (No response.)
> *Therapist*: Could you slide it off the edge of the table or set it on the plate?
> *Child*: (The child makes an independent choice and leans on

the bowl of the spoon with the non-dominant hook and grasps the raised handle with the dominant hook.)

Therapist: Now what do you need to do?

Child: (The child unlocks the elbow and brings the spoon toward her mouth. She attempts to get the spoon in her mouth and pulls the bowl into position.)

Therapist: Is that a good place?

Child: (The child is unsatisfied.)

Therapist: What can you do?

Child: (The child takes spoon in her mouth and lets go with the hook. She attempts to re-grab the spoon but cannot, gets frustrated.)

Therapist: Could you turn your hook so it would grab better?

Child: (The child prepositions the hook with her knees and can grab the handle of the spoon from her mouth successfully.)

Therapist: Will it work now?

Child: (The child moves spoon from mouth to plate successfully using her cable.)

Therapist: That's great! Now shall we try it with food?

It is important to note that parents are encouraged to be present during most treatment sessions. The therapist also spends time educating the parents about the importance of independence and the rationale behind the problem-solving approach to training. The therapist also acts as a role model for the parent to use when carrying out the technique at home.

The same method is used for developing habits of use. As soon as a new skill is mastered, a variety of developmentally appropriate tasks requiring use of that specific skill are introduced and the child is encouraged to master these tasks with as much independence as possible, thus integrating the newly acquired skill into his or her habit patterns. To continue the previous example, the child might be asked to apply make-up, use a fork, or perform simple cooking tasks. The factor of choice in the method of mastery of the task remains primary in the treatment. Suggestions are given only to ensure successful and effective mastery of the task. In some cases, a task selected to encourage use of a new skill may be successfully accomplished without use of that particular skill. This is accepted and the child rewarded for the accomplishment as long as the result is acceptable. Guidelines for acceptability include: that the task is accomplished without undue delay, awkwardness, or energy consumption, and that the result is satisfactory for the developmental level and personal taste of the child. This same approach is used for mastery of activities of daily living whether or not they require use of the prostheses.

This method places the responsibility and success of the program on the skill of the therapist to select tasks which are appropriate for the developmental level and individual interests of the child, and which require the use of the newly acquired skill. Through this process children acquire a history of successful independent problem-solving exprinces both in the mastery of new skills and in the decision-making process of integrating new skills into habits of use. The positive outcome of this approach to treatment is not only children who have mastered use of their prostheses and specific activities of daily living, but also children who, as they mature, are capable and motivated to continue to independently approach unfamiliar tasks and master them.

CASE STUDY

The following case study is presented to illustrate the continued use of a problem-solving approach in the mastery of new skills and habits through adulthood, and the effect an energy deficit has on adaptation to adult roles. It describes the methods of adaptation used by a young woman with multiple limb deficiencies to meet the demands of becoming a competent adult. A brief review of her occupational therapy history describes the historical basis on which her mastery of skills and habits lie. The interview provides a personal account of how she has organized her life to meet her goals and expectations as well as some insight into her perception of the role therapy played in the development of her ability to function as an independent competent adult.

Sue is a 29-year-old Caucasian female. She was originally seen at CAPP at age three years, four months. Her diagnosis at birth was tetrology of Fallot. At three years of age, open heart surgery was performed to correct the defect. Circulatory problems in the extremities developed, resulting in amputation of parts of all four limbs. Her current diagnosis is: quadrilateral amputations—bilateral above-elbow amputations, left below knee amputation, and right partial foot amputation. Her cardiac status is stable with some pulmonary insufficiency, but not enough to affect her current level of function or life span. She is currently fitted with standard body-powered, above-elbow prostheses; a supracondylar, self-suspending, below-knee prosthesis, and a self-suspending, partial-foot prosthesis. She wears all prostheses full waking hours.

Sue has her Masters degree in rehabilitation counseling. She is currently employed three days a week (16 hours) as a Housing and Attendent Referral Specialist at a Center for Independent Living. Sue is married. Her husband Fred is also disabled and uses a powered wheelchair. He is currently employed full-time. They live in a three-bedroom house in the suburbs of a large city in Arizona.

Occupational Therapy History

Sue has always lived in Arizona. Her occupational therapy program was carried out at CAPP on an outpatient basis with the exception of one year of prosthetic training which was carried out in her local commuity under the supervision of the CAPP therapist. By the age of six, Sue had mastered excellent prosthetic skills and spontaneous and appropriate applied use of her prostheses. Therapy was then carried out at semi-annual or annual visits to CAPP and combined with checkout of new prostheses and/or surgical intervention for bony overgrowth of her residual limbs. These visits were usually for one or two weeks. Occupational therapy was carried out as needed to evaluate new prostheses, to familiarize Sue with new prosthetic components, and to assist in mastery of appropriate developmental tasks. Selection of tasks was based on the requests of Sue and her family and on the skill of the therapist to anticipate functional need based on developmental readiness. For example, use of a key had to be mastered before driver's training could begin. Much emphasis was placed on the mastery of desk skills, dressing, and toileting. These tasks could not be mastered at the normal developmental ages because they required a higher level of motivation and prosthetic skill. Parent education was a strong component of the treatment. Because of the limited access to occupational therapy, it was necessary for the parents to be able to recognize appropriate prosthetic use and appropriate expectations for mastery of specific skills. The success of the program depended strongly on the ability of her parents to reward and foster independence in Sue in all aspects of her life. Their support of Sue's efforts to become independent was very important in helping her to develop feelings of competence as an independent individual.

Sue readily mastered independence in eating (with the exception of cutting meat), and desk skills by the age of eight. A swivel spoon was her only necessary piece of adapted equipment. Although dressing was introduced at an early age, full mastery of dressing skills with clothing selected for ease of donning did not occur until 15 years of age. Currently she continues to select clothing for ease of donning and type of fasteners. She uses a button hook and Velcro at the waist of slacks which do not have a belt. Sue also mastered independent toileting and personal hygiene care at age 15. Toileting and personal hygiene are performed without adapted equipment, using only her prostheses.

An independent problem-solving approach to skill acquisition was maintained throughout Sue's selection of the most effective method of completing a task frequently was the most energy efficient. Time was spent with Sue and her family, particularly her mother, explaining and emphasizing the need to set priorities so that energy was available for the more important tasks. A typical example was the suggestion that Sue not be expected to dress herself before school as she needed her time and energy for school work. Undressing at night and dressing on weekends was encouraged to allow adequate practice to develop and maintain these skills.

Regular contact with CAPP was continued until Sue was 21 years of age. At that time, her prosthetic care was shifted to a center nearer her home. Sue still maintains contact with CAPP when a prosthetic problem arises or she has questions about new components or prosthetic designs. She continues to rely on the occupational therapist for adapted equipment (suction cup brush, button hook, and swivel spoon). A conservative estimate of occupational therapy treatment time over the past 26 years would be about 200 hours.

INTERVIEW

The following excerpts from a lengthy interview were selected to illustrate Sue's personal approach to organizing her various adult roles and duties to accommodate both her physical and emotional needs.

Therapist: Let's begin with exploring the effects of your disability on your life style. Do you perceive your life style as being different from that of your friends without disabilities who are in similar life situations?

Sue: Not really, probably more of them have children although we have many single friends. We also have a more casual or less rigid routine to our lives. Work is about the same, but leisure activities are different. We're often too exhausted to do major things after work except eating out, which is actually less work for us than cooking. Therefore we plan weekday leisure activities on the spur of the moment based on our energy levels. We're also less concerned about the appearance of the house—housework in general. If we spent our time to do all the things other people do, could do, or have to do, we wouldn't be able to do anything together. I'm pretty strict about our priorities.

Therapist: How would you list your priorities?

Sue: Probably doing stuff with Fred is number one. Number two is our jobs. His job usually takes priority, it pays more than mine. Then number three is probably responsibilities around the house like laundry. Cooking comes lower than laundry. Even yardwork takes priority for me over cooking. I hate cooking.

Therapist: Do you get assistance with any of these chores?

Sue: Yes, we have a housekeeper once a week and my dad mows the lawn.

Therapist: How would you describe the balance of work, play, and leisure in your life?

Sue: When we are not under stress, they are really well balanced although maybe not typical. Our work schedule is pretty much like anyone else's, employment, that is. Because of my priorities, I reduce the amount of time I spend on household tasks to leave time for leisure activities. These include church activities, time with my family, movies, spectator sports, target practice in the desert, TV. Rest is sometimes a problem. Fred is a night person and we sleep in on the weekends and spend a lazy day in bed to catch up, but that's really leisure too.

Therapist: Your course work in rehabilitation counseling covered crisis theory and the effects described by Selye.[8] Since stress, whether positive or negative, places greater demands on your energy, I would now like to focus on a period of stress in your life to elicit any special efforts you and Fred make to reduce this drain on your energy during these times. Changing jobs is stress producing. What have you and Fred done to cope with this kind of stress?

Sue: When we have new jobs we tend to eat out a lot more, every night for awhile. We are usually exhausted on the weekends and don't do anything, just rest. Things pile up and it takes us time to adjust. Looking at this most recent one with Fred's new job, he got it just 17 days after my grandfather had died.

Therapist: Was your grandfather an important figure in your life?

Sue: Yes, both Fred and I spent time with my grandparents every week at least, especially when Fred was laid off. So we had two things at once and I'm just now getting settled (six months). We weren't getting bills paid, both because of lack of time and lack of money. But when my grandfather was in the hospital, we'd spend a couple of hours there every night, come home, go to bed, a daily routine for three weeks. Mail wasn't even opened. Even though I have a housekeeper things were stacking up and the house was a mess and that's depressing. And then we would only have her clean three days a month to save money and make it worse. That gets me down and until its cleaned up I don't realize why I feel bad. But cleaning house is not a high priority with me.

At first I didn't care that nothing was getting done. And then I began thinking why is this happening and then I began realizing why. I could see it was stress on the new job, and the death, and pressures at my job, and my mom's job, and other family problems related to the death. But things are better now. We're more or less back into our old routines.

Therapist: Even under the tremendous stress of a death in the family, a financial crisis and Fred's new job you've managed to survive and come out intact. To whom or to what do you attribute your abilities to cope with stress, and the fact that you're a competent adult?

Sue: I feel there have been lots of factors. Probably they started at CAPP. Well I know they did and my parents played a big part in it, but they probably wouldn't have played a big part in it without CAPP.

Therapist: Can you describe what it was they did?

Sue: Being free, well, not being over-protected. My mom had to dress me and do extra stuff for me and that did cause some problems between me and my younger siblings and then fighting for me to go to regular school when public school was not something disabled people did. That kind of attitude from them was reinforced by CAPP. They probably stuck with CAPP because its philosophy fit in with the philosophy they felt would work. Probably they supported me and CAPP supported them in an independent philosophy rather than a dependent philosophy.

Working in the disabled community with other disabled persons, you can tell which ones were raised which way and they (the ones who weren't raised to be independent) can't even figure out how to balance a check book! And that to me is inconceivable, I mean I have to teach them how to go out and find a house or an apartment. Nobody taught me how to do it. I mean I was still living at home and I had to go and find an apartment for Fred so he could move out here so we could get married. I found the place myself. I didn't go say "Mommy, I don't know what to do." You go through the paper, find places, and call them up. And you go look at them and see if they're right. Of course sometimes my parents came with me. I wanted a second opinion, but it was I who was going to decide.

I think I manage crises better than Fred. Maybe because I was in the hospital a lot as a kid which was an experience in dealing with recurring crises (15 surgeries for bony overgrowth). I feel like I know how to deal better. In financial crises I don't, I just fall apart. Fred can handle these. He can talk on the phone and tell them this is what we can afford to do. But I can't—don't want to do it.

Therapist: How do you perceive your contact and experiences with occupational therapists contributed to your ability to become an independent and competent adult?

Sue: I never met an occupational therapist I didn't get along with either at CAPP or professionally. They never act superior or dictate what you should do.

Therapist: When you were 15, you spent two days with me working on independence in dressing and household tasks. What did you perceive were the goals of that visit, who did you feel instigated it?

Sue: I don't know, it's hard to answer. I guess intellectually I knew it was time, but I wasn't ready to make the decision myself and it was more like somebody was making me do it.

I really didn't start applying the stuff I learned for another two years. It was stuff I knew how to do and it was great to know how to do it, but for time efficiency's sake, my mom still helped me dress and to this day Fred helps me dress if he has time and the housekeeper changes the sheets even though I can do both tasks. For me, looking back, I knew I would have to, or might have to do that stuff and at least I should know how to do it. Whether I was going to do it or not was another question.

Therapist: What about the philosophy at CAPP, not just independence, but the encouragement of independent problem-solving? In other words, we try not to tell you how to do a task but encourage you to figure it out for yourself. Also we try to show that there is not just one way to do any specific task. Did this get through to you at all?

Sue: Yes, because when you grow up with something like that you don't think about it. But when I was reading over your notes before the interview, and of course I've always observed this, there are people who were disabled later in life or grew up in an atmosphere where they feel there is only one way to do something, and you have to do it that way, and they can't, and therefore they don't do it. For example, I can eat a sandwich with my hooks, but its messy and time consuming so when I'm with my friends or at home, not in public, I just eat it off the plate. One of my coworkers has begun to do the same thing. Up until that time she had always needed to be fed because she can't use her arms. She had never thought about how to figure out how she could eat independently.

Therapist: Finally, if money were no object, what would you change in your current life situation?

Sue: First, a second car, to cut down on daily driving time for me. Second, we would adopt children if we could afford it, and third, I would like a house closer to town, my parents, and church to make socializing with our friends easier by cutting down on driving.

Summary of Case Study

Sue's occupational therapy history reflects an extensive exposure to use of an independent problem-solving approach to mastery of specific tasks as well as considerable counseling of her parents to facilitate a feeling of independence and competence in Sue.

Sue's perception of her current life style reflects a feeling of control and competence in directing her own life. This is typified by her list of priorities. She views her differences from others as stemming from differences in her priorities or financial restrictions. She appears to view her disability as only one aspect of her individuality which affects how she plans her life. Sue's priorities function very effectively to preserve a balance of work, rest, and play in her life. Even under severe stress she is able to step back, re-evaluate and re-establish a balance, noting the reasons for the imbalance as internal reactions to external events.

Sue's perception of the effects and influences of her and her family's exposure to CAPP and to occupational therapy is a combination of a global response to the philosophy of independence and a specific response to memories of experiences in therapy. She identifies the philosophy of independence as being the most important and feels it stems from CAPP's influence on her parents. Her specific response to occupational therapy is one of conflict between maintaining her independence in choosing when and how she will perform certain tasks while intellectually understanding she must master the tasks in order to know that she has the option to perform them independently. The memory of this response occurred at 15 years of age, a critical developmental time for the assertion of independence.

Sue's independent problem-solving skills are so second nature to her that she cannot perceive functioning without them. Her description of how to find an apartment typifies this attitude and illustrates her use of a problem-solving approach to mastery of new tasks as an integral part of her independence.

Finally, she speaks of how her life style would be if it were free of financial limitations. The major task identified as making her current life style different from her married friends is not having children. She also lists two solutions to the current major drain on her energy, driving. It is clear that Sue perceives herself as capable of assuming all the necessary roles of adulthood for her choice of life style.

She feels confident that through setting priorities her limitations due to her amputations, especially her energy deficit, can be compensated for and will not hinder her in achievement of her life goals.

SUMMARY

An independent problem-solving approach to mastery of skills and habits has been proposed as a method of aiding children with multiple limb deficiencies to develop mastery of prosthetic skills and activities of daily living. It was further suggested that the development of these problem-solving skills assist in forming a history which continues to support their abilities to independently master the changing developmental skills and habits necessary to continue to function competently throughout the life cycle.

The case study of a young woman illustrated the successful accomplishment of excellent prosthetic operating skills and applied use of the prostheses as well as mastery of the major activities of daily living. It also illustrated how, as an adult, she incorporated an independent problem-solving approach into mastery of skills and habits necessary for a competent performance of adult roles. It is important to note that her energy deficit was the portion of her disability which required her to use the greatest levels of problem-solving and adaptation to accommodate to adult role demands. In CAPP's experience it appears that the development of a problem-solving approach to mastery of skills and habits early in childhood, in order to establish a history of positive experiences in problem-solving behavior, will continue to nurture competence and efficacy throughout the life cycle.

REFERENCES

1. Montgomery M: Resources of adaptation for daily living: Classification with therapeutic implications for occupational therapy. *Occup Ther Health Care,* 4:9-23, 1984

2. Frank G: Life history model of adaptation to disability: The case of a congenital amputee. *Soc Sci Med* (19)6:639-645, 1984

3. Setoguchi Y, Rosenfelder R: The Limb Deficient Child. Springfield: Thomas Publishers, 1982

4. CAPP—University of California at Los Angeles Child Amputee Prosthetics Project. First Annual Report, 1955

5. Elkind D: Child Development and Education, A Piagetian Perspective. New York: Oxford Press, 1976

6. Kielhofner G, Burke J: A model of human occupation, Part 1. Conceptual framework and content. *Am J Occu Ther* (34)9:577-579, 1980

7. Lee T, Magill R: The locus of contextual interference in motor-skill acquisition. *J Exp Psychol,* 4:730-746, 1983

8. Selye H: Stress Without Distress. New York: Harper and Row, Inc. 1974

Using Purpose
to Engage the Patient
With Depression

Andrea Davis-Kosaka, OTR
Deborah Kraml, OTR
Shawn Miyake, MA, OTR
Colleen Rochford, OTR

ABSTRACT. At the very heart of occupational therapy practice is the active engagement of the patient with purposeful activities. The lack of energy displayed by some psychiatric patients is often viewed by occupational therapists as a barrier to the very treatment process they are trying to implement. When patients fail to participate in treatment, therapists are often frustrated and confused about what steps to take next. This paper will examine the process of involving low-energy psychiatric patients in activity across four dimensions: imparting purpose, the role of choice, meeting expectations and interaction with peers. Treatment implications are outlined and discussed in respect to three case studies.

Occupational therapy has always placed a significant importance upon, if not been dependent on, the patient's active engagement in his treatment.[1,2] In occupational therapy practice, therapists are concerned with eliciting the patient's participation in the treatment process.[2] The process of occupational therapy addresses the remediation of dysfunctional states by the active engagement of the patient in "purposeful activities."[3] "Issues of major concern in this therapeutic approach are a patient's willingness to engage in the activity, the value that is attached by patients to participating in the ac-

Andrea Davis-Kosaka is staff occupational therapist, adolescent services; Deborah Kraml is staff occupational therapist, adult services; Shawn Miyake is director of Adjunctive Therapy; Colleen Rochford is staff occupational therapist, young adult services; all are on staff at Woodview Calabasas Hospital, 25100 Calabasas Road, Calabasas, CA 91302.

This article appears jointly in *Occupational Therapy for the Energy Deficient Patient* (The Haworth Press, 1986) and *Occupational Therapy in Health Care*, Volume 3, Number 1 (Spring 1986).

41

tivity, and the future use of skills that are developed in the process."[2:254] In short, the patient must hold a reason or purpose to initiate involvement in the treatment.

Of major frustration to occupational therapists practicing in psychiatry is the 'energy deficient' patient who has been diagnosed as depressed. For purposes of this paper, such a patient will be referred to as someone who displays a low energy level.[4] This low energy level is present in most depressed persons and is observed even in the absence of demand for physical activity.[4] Combined with a sense of worthlessness and hopelessness, these patients prove to be very difficult to engage in activity. Entire staffs are frustrated to the point of literally dumping such patients out of bed in an attempt to get them involved in 'something.'

In this paper, composite descriptions of three patients at an acute inpatient psychiatric facility who display typical poor engagement in therapeutic program will be examined. These cases are drawn from adolescent, young adult and adult populations. Each bears a diagnostic label of major depression. Similarities and differences in their characteristics and management will be discussed across four dimensions:

I. *Imparting Purpose*—How is meaning or value of an activity translated and integrated into a patient's perceived sense of values?

II. *The Role of Choice*— How does a patient view choice in purposeful activity in a therapeutic environment?

III. *Meeting Expectations*—Whose needs are being met and what purpose is served when the low energy patient is encouraged to participate?

IV. *Interaction With Peers*—In what way does peer support facilitate the low-energy patient to find meaning in activity?

These dimensions of activity planning and use appear clinically relevant when working with the depressed, low-energy person and are reflective of needs shown in the diagnostic features of depression.[4]

CASE EXAMPLES

Case One—CK

CK is a 13 year old female admitted to the hospital following a suicide attempt. CK's parents were divorced when she was four years old at which time she received counseling periodically for about three years. During this period CK lived with her mother and was able to maintain her role as a student. Two or three months prior to the current admission, discord between CK and her mother increased. CK had requested to have counseling again but her mother denied her need for it even though CK's school grades had begun to slide from A's and B's to C's and D's. She was also truant from most of her classes and became gradually isolated and withdrawn from friends and family members. CK began to experience recurrent sleep disturbances, uncontrolled anger and an inability to control outbursts of rage toward her mother. Just prior to admission, CK and her mother had had a heated argument regarding their possible relocation to another city. This proved to be intolerable to CK and resulted in a suicide attempt and the present hospitalization.

Upon admission, CK was observed to be emotionally labile. Sudden mood swings were common. As occupational therapy evaluation ascertained that she was unable to initiate involvement in what were prior interests, e.g., sewing and sports. She frequently complained of boredom, uselessness and 'feeling run down,' which interfered with her ability to attend school regularly and pursue leisure interests. It was also found her frustration tolerance was poor due to her inability to recognize obstacles and match requisite skills to realistic goals. For instance, CK had accepted part-time employment for which she did not possess adequate skills, taking on the responsibility of babysitting without experience or help in learning what it required.

In the hospital CK was placed in both the occupational therapy workshop and leisure education program to encourage participation in past interests and to develop some leisure options. In addition, in a life skills group she participated in a prevocational module to encourage more realistic development of future goals based on both current and future attainable skills.

Case Two—JW

JW is a twenty year old male who was admitted to the hospital following a suicide attempt. In interview in occupational therapy he stated that over the last year he had been feeling progressively worse, that prior to then 'things were O.K.' He reported having recently graduated from high school where he was a 'B' student. Although he engaged in extracurricular activities he would not describe himself as one of the popular boys. He also reported having comforting, supportive but overly protective parents. He was not allowed to date until his junior year of high school and was discouraged from working part-time during his senior year. After graduation JW decided to live at home while attending junior college and working part-time at a clothing store. JW began to date more frequently during this time and became seriously involved with a woman at work who was several years older than he. As their relationship progressed JW began using drugs on a daily basis. Ignoring his parents' displeasure, JW moved out of the family home and in with his girlfriend. He states, "this was the beginning of the end." His relationship with his parents became strained, he began distancing himself from peers at school and work and became increasingly dependent on his girlfriend. After five months, the relationship with his girlfriend ended. JW chose to keep his apartment and juggle his hectic school and work schedules. In time, he quit school to concentrate on work. He became financially dependent on his parents, stopped seeing friends, discontinued participation in previous leisure interests, and escalated his abuse of marijuana. Following several warnings at work and continued poor work performance, JW was fired, at which point he attempted suicide.

Upon admission, JW described himself as feeling "sad and down, helpless and hopeless, and unable to cope with life." The occupational therapy evaluation revealed deficits in the area of money management which reinforced his dependency on his family and girlfriend. His inability to manage his time effectively eroded his performance at school and work, ultimately resulting in his dismissal. JW was placed in a life skills program to improve his independent living skills, particularly in time and money management. He was also involved in a variety of leisure task groups to provide him with leisure options.

JW found it increasingly difficult to attend occupational therapy groups and when there, could not initiate any tasks stating "I can't do it" or "I'm too tired."

Case Three—DR

DR is a fifty year old widow. She describes an extended depression with the feeling that life "is not worth living." She reports a loss of appetite and difficulty sleeping. Although she was unable to identify the onset of the current episode, it appears to relate to the beginning of the illness and subsequent death from cancer of her husband of 30 years. DR describes that although her husband was able to accept his impending death, she denied it constantly. After an initial period of grieving she was able to live alone in her home. As the days went on, however, DR gradually began to lose her motivation to perform day-to-day tasks and started to let things 'slide.' She began to isolate herself and became increasingly unhappy. She believed that she was no longer capable of managing herself or her home. DR subsequently moved in with her 25 year old son and his family.

DR's history includes a hospitalization some 20 years previously for depression and family history also reveals she had an alcoholic father who died when she was 15 years old and a mother who committed suicide five years after that. It was at about that time that DR married and had a son. She has therefore maintained the role of a housewife since the age of twenty and has had few leisure interests outside of the home.

Upon admission, DR was observed to be tearful and preoccupied with a sense of hopelessness and helplessness. She is fearful she will never get well, questions the value of continuing her life and is unable to engage in a task, stating, ''I'm too old'' and ''I'm just a burden.'' The occupational therapy evaluation disclosed prior succsssful role enactment as a homemaker until the death of her husband. The patient was unable, however, to indicate involvement in any leisure interests except for activities which revolved around the homemaker role. With her husband gone, DR is unable to see the value of the activities in which she previously engaged. She spends much of her time in isolation.

DR was placed in a cooking group to regain appreciation for the socially and personally satisfying aspects of the activity apart from the perception of simply fulfilling a duty as in her previous role. She was also involved in various communication groups to facilitate interaction with peers and discussion of issues relative to making role transitions in later life. DR's involvement in the occupational therapy workshop, both in small groups and alone, encouraged the development of leisure interests.

ENGAGING THE PATIENT: A CROSS CASE COMPARISON

The persons in all three cases presented share the diagnostic label of depression. They are similar to each other in symptoms presented, which are characteristic of depression.[4,5] They are different from each other because they are unique individuals who have distinct histories, interests, values and tasks relevant to their developmental periods in life. Of concern here, however, is the similar difficulty found in engaging each patient in activity. Staff believe the occupational therapy process depends on the idea that a patient engage in some purposeful acitivity, i.e., one that has a meaning attached to it by each patient,[3] that will ultimately facilitate treatment, the achievement of goals and behavioral change. But what happens when the patient is unwilling to accede to the therapist's purpose for doing the activity and thus fails to participate in the treatment? This issue of engagement will be examined across the following four dimensions: imparting purpose, the role of choice, meeting expectations and interaction with peers.

Imparting Purpose

Inherent in the process of occupational therapy is the idea that there is purpose for the participation of the patient in an activity or task. Although the therapeutic value of such participation may be clear to the therapist who selects it, it may not be so to the patient. The three cases illustrate this potential problem.

In *CK's* situation it was difficult to relate the purpose of activity to her because of her resistance or inability to focus on *any* future goals or plans. Her response to an explanation of a craft activity's purpose was "what's the point? I really don't think doing any of these things will make me feel any better." She was unable to focus on any aspects of her life, other than her immediate feelings which prevented her from anticipating any future gain from participation in the craft activity. There was no inherent satisfaction in participating in the task or value placed on learning skill components within the task, despite the fact that the craft activity (sewing was chosen) was both a past interest of hers and one in which she had some successful experiences.

Initially, *JW* had difficulty waking in the morning and attending any groups, but within several days he was attending groups with the encouragement of staff. Once in group, the occupational therapist explained the purpose of the life skills group with its focus on competencies necessary to function within roles and the current difficulties individuals in the group might be having maintaining adequate role performance. JW stated that he had all the skills he needed and that the only problem he had was that he lost his job.

This he said would all be taken care of when he got out of the hospital and found another job. In the occupational therapy workshop, JW found it difficult to understand why he had to do apparently "unrelated craft projects." He furthermore, could not relate any of the activities in the occupational therapy workshop or life skills group to his attempt at taking his life.

DR had difficulty seeing the value of any activity that was now outside of her lost housewife role. She found it useless to engage in activities or projects that would not be applicable to maintaining the home and caring for a spouse. The end of her role as a housewife following her husband's death was also the loss of her main source of self-fulfillment and self-satisfaction. Leisure activities held no place of value to her as they had no place in her former role. Thus, participation in the occupational therapy workshop was difficult for her.

Summary and Intervention: In all three cases, the potential value that various activities hold for the patients is lost to them due to depressive illness; they see little purpose for engagement in anything. Furthermore, any attempt at imparting purpose is met by stiff resistance on the patient's part despite the fact that skill components, interests and values involved did relate to past valued roles, and current and future plans were addressed. Often, patients will voice difficulty with engaging in tasks even though they agree to the apparent usefulness of such activities in their current situations, i.e., regaining worker role behaviors by attending life skills groups. The environment and demands to which patients will return must be discussed with them in order to establish levels of mutual understanding. Only then can the goals of the therapist and patient be shared and translated into a program that can be implemented. The patient's reality can be addressed in such a discussion while at the same time the therapist's goals are explained in light of the patient's current situation. In this way, the patient may come to view the therapist's goals as assisting him to meet his own goals for hospitalization.

In *CK's* case, this means one must address her immediate feelings of hopelessness. The patient states that she just wants to feel in control of her life. This need is not so far from the therapist's goals of assisting her toward task accomplishment and mastery. When these ideas are compared, the patient is able to see that the goals are quite similar. The concrete feedback that a patient receives from success in appropriately chosen activities in the occupational therapy workshop demonstrates and reinforces the feeling that one *can* have an effect on his own environment. From this realization a sense of self-respect and an attitude of hopefulness toward the world can be cultivated.[6]

In *JW's* case, a similar process may be attempted with the addition of graded involvement in a life skills group. The patient may be encouraged to sit and listen to others during the activity or read pertinent material. The use of peer models who have experienced similar situations and who are attempting to take risks and make decisions that may alter the course of their present circumstances may also prove useful in identifying the relevance of this activity to real life situations. The constant feedback by both staff and peers regarding the relationship of lifeskill tasks and their functional everyday counterparts builds up the patient's sense of purpose in his involvement in the task.

In *DR's* case, a mutual exploration of her changed role would prove useful. Unfilled goals of life may be addressed in a rethinking of her current role. In this case, the patient has always had the desire to serve persons less fortunate than herself. Combined with her many caregiving and homemaker skills, a successful transition into volunteer work serving disabled persons meets her needs and allows her to engage in previously satisfying activities.

In all three cases, the respectful and close attention that is paid to the patients as they discuss their realities communicates more than a sense of warmth and acceptance. It strengthens a patient's sense of competency, thus reinforcing their perception that they can influence their environment. In broader terms, this can be translated by patients into a perspective that they have value and self-worth because of their ability to influence the environment and can thus develop much needed self-respect. To the low-energy, depressed patient who sees no purpose in life in general, his ability to have a meaningful effect upon the human and non-human environment reinforces an active, coping orientation to life as opposed to a passive, hopeless attitude.[6,7]

Role of Choice

The role of choice in the engagement process involves both the patient and the therapist. Patients are usually given the opportunity to choose an activity that fits within personal interests and mutually defined treatment goals. Although an activity may be intrinsically motivating to a patient, the focus can be adapted by the therapist to address certain issues, e.g., an interest in solitary listening to music may be redirected to small group music listening and sharing about music groups.

From the very start, *CK* was unwilling to assume any responsibility for making choices. Her passive and submissive behavior was a source of frustration to staff and peers alike. Her typical response was, "well I guess your idea is good, never mind mine." Any choices that she made were only accepted on the basis of peer or staff approval. Prior experiences in which she was unable to control certain outcomes, e.g., mother denying her requests for therapy and planning to move away, all contributed to her feelings of helplessness and hopelessness. From the occupational therapy evaluation it became apparent that CK had never developed a sense of efficacy based on prior experiences.

In a similar way, *JW* chose passively to attend an activity, but he clothed his approach to acceptance in a false competency in which he waived off any attempts at activity engagement or offered choice because he apparently 'had everything together.' Most tasks were of no interest because they were 'obviously too simple' or he 'already knew how to do it.' In the occupational therapy workshop, although presented with many choices, he was unable to make up his mind. He continued to maintain his facade of competence. When finally pushed to make a choice between two selected projects, he would choose the easier of the two stating, "it really didn't matter" and in this way he diffused any potential risk of failure or incompetency.

DR's situation was different from the previous two examples in that she saw all choices as a waste of time and meaningless. This put her into a double bind and produced much frustration within her, because she could not see the purpose in any choice and since she was not making a choice, she interpreted this as evidence of her worthlessness and incompetence.

Summary and Intervention: It is often the case that when a patient makes no choice, then this decision becomes the choice itself. No choice is in essence a choice not to participate. While on the surface this may appear to be a passive and submissive action, it is not without purpose. To make a choice to act is possibly to confront the very incompetence the patient anxiously avoids. Because so few choices are made and those that may have been carried out have resulted in failure experiences, the patient has few action strategies from which to choose. Those at their disposal have either negative or non-existent feedback attached to them.[7] When a patient is able to successfully negotiate an activity or task, he thereby refines his strategies for achieving an objective. The patient also builds a competent self-image capable of examining the realities of action choices and the boundaries of reasonable objectives.[7]

In all three cases cited, the lack of choice can be traced to the need to avoid incompetence. In the first two cases, CK and JW avoid performing to escape expected incompetence. In the case of DR she avoids demonstrating to herself the worthlessness of her decisions. This kind of issue can be approached in the following way. All three patients are invited to investigate the variety of projects available to them. Of those offered, two or three are identified by the therapist as feasible on the basis of voiced interest, potential for high degree of success and short-term or immediate gratification of task. The activity that is the 'perceived choice' of the patient is then given to him. Expectations for participation are kept at a minimal level and are clearly voiced. In time, with small successes, additional tasks, graded upward, can be used.

Meeting Expectations

Occupational therapists are often excited by the observed increase in participation of a previously low-energy inactive patient. What very rarely crosses the mind of the therapist is the thought, "for whom is the patient doing the task?" Many therapists only consider this after hearing a patient comment to a passerby, "I'm only doing this because they said to do it."

CK attempted to meet all expectations of her peers, staff and family. She participated in the occupational therapy workshop projects because she believed that her involvement would result in staff approval. When given choices, her typical response was, "you choose, you know what's best for me."

As JW became more involved in his treatment, he began to rely on the "level system" in place on the unit. This system is a behavioral reward system that encourages patient participation and responsibility in their treatment. JW performed the necessary behaviors that would maintain his present "level." His typical remarks would include such statements as, "if this is what you want me to do, then I'll do it." JW consistently asked for staff feedback regarding progress on tasks, failing to trust his own sense of accomplishment.

Like JW, *DR* constantly sought out the therapist's feedback to "make sure" that she was doing the task "right." She constantly remarked, "I hope that I am doing it the way I'm supposed to." Her attendance in the occupational therapy workshop was tied into the granting of her passes and became the sole reason for attendance there.

Summary and Intervention: When one's accomplishments and sense of effectiveness is verified and given value by others, one's sense of value as a human being is confirmed.[7] A patient's sense of personal value in self and in an activity is derived in part from the feedback that he receives from others. Feedback from others verifies to the patient that something has been learned or accomplished, and that such is of value to others. Self-esteem evolves from the intrinsic gratification of the accomplishment and the feedback from others about the accomplishment.[7]

In all of the cases, as was previously discussed, the therapist could take the time to discuss with the patient what expectations each has regarding the outcome of the activity. In this way, the patient's and the therapist's expectations for performance are compared and clarified. Initially, direct feedback regarding performance may be given by the therapist until the patient can begin to respond to questions regarding his own performance, e.g., "what do you think of the result of your action?", "what could you have done differently?", "what do you think the next step might be?" Such questions allow the patient to safely try out his thoughts about his own skill and ability to meet life's challenges.[2]

Interaction With Peers

The interaction with peers is an important arena within which one can attempt, compare and adjust action strategies.

CK assumed a passive stance in relation to her peers. She socialized with them by merely being in their presence. Her participation in activities relied upon their positive feedback. When given negative feedback, she became sullen and angered. She verbally denigrated her peers and any stuctured activity. Her peers supported her helplessness by making choices for her or completing projects for her at her request.

When *JW* was finally able to attend groups, he maintained a passive interaction with staff, only responding to their questions and never generating any of his own. He did not initiate any conversation with peers. The assertiveness of his peers in the group only served to make him isolate himself more. Other young adult patients who had entered the hospital under similar circumstances offered JW support. JW appeared to be afraid of making a connection with any of his peers and risk possible rejection from them. When encouraged by staff to attempt interacting with patients on the unit, he stated that he 'didn't want any friends from a psychiatric hospital,' but was soon observed sitting with others who were known as depressed and who had been offering their support to him.

In *DR's* case, interaction with peers encouraged her participation in activities and tasks. Although she was reluctant to make a choice about anything, she did join a group of patients who were about two or three steps ahead of her in the treatment process.

Summary and Intervention: In the best of milieu treatment settings, peers emerge as a major treatment influence. They are "models who exemplify competent responses to the problems of adaptation that the (patient) faces (and) have a potentially dual significance. They aid (patients) in discovering what they need to do to succeed in their task, to solve their problems. But they also can give them realistic grounds for hope, particularly when the model is another similarly situated (patient) who is a step or so further along in the therapeutic process."[6:15] In occupational therapy groups, the therapist, but more importantly the peer group, can become a major force in motivating the patient. The patient tends to operate from a singular base, that no one can ever relate to his present feelings of hopelessness and incompetence.

As in DR's situation, peers proved to be the encouraging factor. They got her involved in the first step, that of attending the group. Peers serve as a support. They can share purpose with a patient by discussing the value and benefits of participation in an activity. They also serve as role models for others to see that engagement is acceptable, that others can value their work or involvement. Peers can promote socialization and expression of issues and feelings, all in a subtly therapeutic way that staff intervention could probably never accomplish.

SUMMARY

The lack of response of depressed, low-energy patients in all treatment settings proves to be a major obstacle to occupational therapy programming. In psychiatric settings, patient participation in activity is viewed as the very core of the therapeutic process. When patients fail to value and find therapeutic meaning in tasks and activities placed before them, a closer examination of purpose is necessary. The use of purpose in engagement of the low-energy patient with depression has been discussed across four dimensions: imparting purpose, the role of choice, meeting expectations and interaction with peers. Similarities and differences in attention to these elements were discussed in relation to three cases and treatment implications were outlined.

Although no final answers about engaging patients in tasks can be drawn from these illustrations, the process of therapeutic engagement may be summed up in the thoughts of Adolph Meyer, "Our role consists in giving opportunities rather than prescriptions. There are no royal roads; it is all a problem of being true to one's nature and opportunities and of teaching others to do the same with themselves. It takes a resourcefulness and ability to respect the native capacities and interests of the patients. With this background we will be able to shape for our patients and ourselves an outlook of sound idealism, furnishing a setting within which apparently insurmountable difficulties will be conquered."[8]

REFERENCES

1. Florey L: Intrinsic motivation: The dynamics of occupational therapy theory. *Am J Occup Ther,* 23:4, 319-322, 1969

2. Burke J: A clinical perspective on motivation: Pawn vs origin. *Am J Occup Ther,* 31:4, 254-258, April, 1977

3. Position Paper on Purposeful Activities, American Occupational Therapy Association, Commission on Practice. Adopted April, 1983 by Representative Assembly

4. *Diagnostic and Statistical Manual of Mental Disorders,* 3rd ed., American Psychiatric Association, Washington, D.C., 1980

5. Goodwin DW and Guze SB: *Psychiatric Diagnosis,* 2nd ed., Oxford University Press, New York, 1979

6. Brewster Smith M: Competence and adaptation. *Am J Occup Ther,* 28:1, 11-15, January, 1974

7. Fidler GS and Fidler JW: Doing and becoming: Purposeful action and self-actualization. *Am J Occup Ther,* 32:5, 305-319, May-June, 1978

8. Meyer A: The Philosophy of Occupation Therapy. *Arch Occ Ther* 1, 1-10, 1922

Psychic Energy—The Activator of the Low Energy Patient

Doris Fredericka Rosenbusch, MA, OTR

ABSTRACT. The article presents a description of a theoretical basis for how psychic energy can be harnessed to activate the low energy patient to physical performance which otherwise would be unobtainable. It shows how this vitalizer varies with each individual and how it varies over time for one individual. A longitudinal case study, in log form, illustrates the progression of change in one patient at various levels of diminished physical energy and performance. For the occupational therapist treating patients with difficult restorable clinical symptoms and/or poor prognosis, psychic energy and its potentials is seen as a useful tool.

If a human being has suffered the tragic indignity of becoming a biological wreck from whatever cause, how does that individual fight back? What ignites him or her to take action against the incredible odds of the almost impossible? And if that recovery takes years or if the condition is long term lasting until death, what energizes him or her to continue the struggle. Assuming that one had personal health and a vital life before the onslaught of the physical disease or accident, the answer appears to be healthy psychic energy.

THE NATURE OF PSYCHIC ENERGY

Freud states in an original 1910 lecture on the *The Origin and Development of Psycho-Analysis,* "The energetic and successful man is he who succeeds by dint of labour in transforming his wish

Doris Fredericka Rosenbusch received her occupational therapy degrees from Eastern Michigan University and the University of Southern California. Her private practice office is at 3763 Inglewood Blvd., Los Angeles, CA 90066.

This article appears jointly in *Occupational Therapy for the Energy Deficient Patient* (The Haworth Press, 1986) and *Occupational Therapy in Health Care,* Volume 3, Number 1 (Spring 1986).

55

fancies into reality."[1,p.18] Or as Arieti words it, "Moreover, what appear to us as conscious phenomena are only the last steps of a long series of unconscious processes. For instance, a thought or a complicated movement of our hands is the end result of a very long chain of mechanisms, of which only the terminal ones reach consciousness."[2,p.17] Awareness introduces into reality the factor of the psyche, its energy, and its capability to effect difficult changes. Awareness affects the individual's inner homeostatic equilibrium. An inner imbalance causes psychic pain or discomfort. The individual finds it important to remove this pain or discomfort, which creates a need.[2]

THE NEED FOR DIGNITY

Daily, in my twenty-six year old private practice of treating long term physical recovery patients (up to eight years in duration with some) I observe the very real phenomenon of psychic energy. Healthy psychic energy in the individuals I treat is that need which looks for and finds inner dignity in a condition lacking outward dignity. Dignity is somehow brought to this moment of life experience not just by the awareness of the moment but by personal awareness of the 'universality' of the moment. The real or symbolic awareness of the universality of life's experiences is realized in such events as birth, growth, fruition, creativity, enjoyment, love, discovery, recovery, decay, and death. The universality of events of the moment is not just for human beings but exists in all forms of nature. And for man, it also exists in his awareness of his influence upon other human beings and upon nature; and as Searles wrote, his awareness of his subjective unity with the manmade environment.[3]

HOW TO ENERGIZE PSYCHIC ENERGY

To quote Frankel, "For the meaning of life differs from man to man, from day to day, and from hour to hour. What matters, therefore, is not the meaning of life in general but rather the specific meaning of a person's life at a given moment."[4,p.171] Universal awareness changes from moment to moment and takes many forms of expression. Different expressions ignite individual's psychic strengths differently, energizing them to actively overcome physical infirmity. Some of the expressions which might vitalize the psyche are:

1. humor/wit/comedy which gives one self-detachment from suffering;
2. deliberate attention to the wind/rain/sun/shade/sunsets, or to the ticking/chiming of a clock or to any phenomenon which helps the individual somatosensorially or symbolically experience the passing of time;
3. deliberate placement in one's immediate environment of unusual or exotic plants such as an amaryllis bulb, an orchid or gloxinia flower, a bonsai tree, a terrarium garden or any object of nature which conveys the message that the unusual is usual in nature;
4. anecdotal stories, pictures, movies, or real observations about bird/butterfly/dog/cat behavior, especially about how these creatures respond to having a fracture/amputation/genetic deficit, or any adaptive behavior to a limitation, or any event which gives understanding of how graded and gradual changes occur during restoration;
5. conversation about how an individual's suffering can provide learning and assist with medical research or the advancement of medical knowledge;
6. the anticipation of or a true sharing of a moment with a loved one, or any dedication to a cause greater then oneself;
7. any relationship to a creative art, such as painting/photography/ sculpture/literature/drama/music/crafts, which symbolizes or tells of unique yet 'universal' experiences i.e., French Impressionist or American Scene paintings, photography collections as in the books *The Family of Man* and *The Family of Children,* Rodin sculptures, O. Henry short stories, Verdi operas, Andrew Lloyd Weber's Requiem mass, Beethoven's music, or/ and primitive craft objects; and
8. the study or discussion of collected knowledge of civilization in any of the many hundreds of books on such subjects as history/poetry/religion/philosophy/psychology/astronomy/anthropology, or any subject which enlightens the individual's understanding of the life experience.

During therapy any of these expressions of psychic energy can be incorporated with physical disability treatment or made part of the treatment milieu.

ROLE OF PSYCHIC ENERGY

Many individuals with very low physical energy spend the majority of their day in psychic energy pursuits. When physical energy or performance increases psychic energy expressions appear to remain as initiators of physical activity but frequently become secondary or equal in allotted time. Also, the psychic energy expressions change over the course of time thus providing different kinds and qualities of stimuli. These initiators sometimes surface showing a direct relationship to actual treatment modalities but sometimes they remain as a subtle inner motivation to the general drive for life and health.

To illustrate the theory, the following case study is presented. Mrs. J. F., a lady in her sixties, was treated by me in her home three times weekly for three years. She suffered a cerebral vascular accident on April 1, 1978, and was initially seen on April 11, 1978. Her hemiplegia involved the left side of her body but this was not her most disabling condition. What kept her bed-ridden or homebound for three years was hypostatic and labile blood pressure. The sensation on the left side was hyper. The goal of treatment in occupational therapy was to restore her left upper extremity from zero strength to any functional performance possible, while avoiding the development of spasticity.

The following double diary account extracted from treatment records shows the important changes in her physical condition along with changes in psychic expression as they occurred over time. Some forms of the psychic energy directly connect to treatment progress or modalities and some remain as inner motivating forces. The first column gives the posting of time; the second column shows the general category number of one or more of the forms of psychic expression (listed in prior section above); the third column describes the specific individualization of Mrs. J.F.'s psychic expressions; and the fourth column presents significant changes in her physical conditions.

TIME Dates:	Form #	PSYCHIC EXPRESSIONS	PHYSICAL CONDITIONS
6-30-78	2	Mrs. J.F. had a strong bond with nature and watched the passing of the day from her bedroom window especially the sun/shade/wind on the trees and flowers.	The first use of her left hand was the holding of several medium sized jam jars and repeatedly taking the tops off and putting them on with her right hand.

TIME		PSYCHIC EXPRESSIONS	PHYSICAL CONDITIONS
Dates:	Form #		
7-1-78 to 7-30-78	4	Then her elderly pet dog suddenly got sick and died, and she transferred her feelings to the therapist's pet dog who was suffering from a heart condition.	Twice a day for several hours at a time she sat up in bed.
7-31-78	2	She spent fifteen minutes in her livingroom in order to watch the evening sunset.	Her total wheelchair sitting tolerance was fifteen minutes.
8-12-78	3	Gifts of exotic flower arrangements were sent to her from family and friends; she was still too weak for their visits.	With her left hand, using pad pinches she was able to hold light weight objects: a small coin purse, a cosmetic case, her compact and a plum. She started having therapy in the livingroom— wheelchair tolerance, one hour.
8-31-78	4	The major topic of conversation during therapy was the relationships of her two pet parrots to the wild birds (sometimes injured ones) that were in her patio just outside the livingroom glass doors.	This day she peeled a banana with her left hand.
10-13-78	1	A humorous therapeutic relationship began because of her frankness about the dullness of the therapy regimen.	She held a peach with her left hand while cutting it in half with her other hand; also, carried a sweater over her left arm while walking twenty steps with a cane.
10-16-78	7	By college education she was a social worker, but by nature a person interested in many aspects of artistic, creative, and cultural human developments.	She combined a gross grip with left arm reaching movements in the functional activity of washing her right full arm and hand. Carried a book in her left bent arm, and later in the day started reading it.

TIME Dates:	Form #	PSYCHIC EXPRESSIONS	PHYSICAL CONDITIONS
10-23-78	6	For two months getting ready for Christmas was her main stimulator. She was anticipating the joy of being with her husband, three adult children, and two grandchildren. Her purchase of gifts was by mail order.	To wrap the gifts she started tying large bows bilaterally by using a left lateral pinch. Also, she was trying to use a light grip in wringing out a washcloth.
4-6-79	1	A humorous birthday gift to me was the joke of the day.	She wrapped this gift, bilaterally, using wrapping paper, elastic cord and a bow.
7-2-79	8	Her main topic of conversation was about her life travels and her understanding of these cultural experiences.	Total wheelchair tolerance has increased to four hours. She held a nail file in her left hand between the thumb and index finger while filing the nails of the other hand.
	6	Daily she played for at least two hours either Rummy Tile, Scrabble, or Mah-Jongg with her husband.	
8-10-79	2	Enjoyment of the sun and water noticeably energized her.	While standing in her backyard swimming pool she developed some bilateral arm stroke movements.
9-21-79	6	She was stimulated by finding creative solutions to the everyday enjoyment of cooking for and eating dinner with her husband; also, in teaching him how to do microwave oven cooking.	Using her left hand to hold many different objects she prepared some foods in the kitchen from her wheelchair.
11-26-79	6	More and more she spoke of her enjoyment of the visits with her life-long friends.	Her left hand held a two ounce can while operating the electric can opener.
12-11-79	6	Again, her planning and preparing for Christmas fireside festivities dominated her time.	She held the end of a purse zipper, using a left pad pinch, while opening her purse.

TIME		PSYCHIC EXPRESSIONS	PHYSICAL CONDITIONS
Dates:	Form #		
1-16-80	4	Her joy was in bringing into her home a new pet, a dog guide for the blind, who could no longer do the job due to a chronic stomach condition.	She filed her nails using the more difficult action of a left pad pinch in contrast to the previous lateral pinch.
2-17-80 to 2-24-80	1	Her sense of humor was her constant forte.	Mrs. J.R. was hospitalized for a basilar artery (bilateral) stroke giving her double vision, vertigo, slurring of speech, and bilateral muscle weakness and tightness.
2-25-80 to 7-27-80	4, 1, 8, 3, 6	Her vitalizers were the relationship to her dog, her humorous nature, a psychologist's radio talk-show, exotic indoor plants, and the verbal jumblegrams and crossword puzzles she played with her husband.	Due to her constant labile blood pressure she was bed-ridden for five months. She learned how to work the tape recorder and talking books on loan from the Braille Institute.
7-28-80	6	She began the planning for and then supervising of the workmen for two major household restorations: a special fireproof roof and the resurfacing of all the hardwood floors.	She ate her first meal sitting at a table in the livingroom during the sunset hour.
9-15-80	6	Being able to eat her meals with her husband again was a great joy for her.	The making of simple salads and tuna salad sandwiches became her bilateral hand functions.
11-27-80	6	She was still determined to work on home restoration jobs along with her own restoration.	The project of making the turkey dressing for her family Thanksgiving Day celebration was totally her work.
12-29-80	6 & 2	During December she enjoyed the Christmas gatherings along with the Pacific ocean red winter sunsets.	Her daily wheelchair tolerance became nine hours.

TIME		PSYCHIC EXPRESSIONS	PHYSICAL CONDITIONS
Dates:	Form #		
2-12-81	5	Conversation during therapy was mainly about the current medical knowledge concerning her condition and her husband's need for hip replacement surgery.	She washed her own hair using both hands/arms and did her own nail care.
3-29-81	7	The major topic of conversation was about different cultures and the artistic objects she had collected in her lifetime of travels.	She began learning about, and then working bilaterally on, a gross stitch needlepoint pillow project.
5-12-81	6	Delighted by the colorful and lively helium balloons given to her on Mother's Day her mood was buoyant.	Daily she worked on her needlepoint for two hours.
Memorial Day Weekend 1981			Friday Mrs. J.F. suffered her third stroke and died that night.

SUMMARY AND CONCLUSIONS

In summary, physical energy is not vitalized to physical performance in and of itself. Its catalyst is psychic energy. As a therapist, you can help your patient find and direct the healthy psychic energy which needs to be tapped if physical rehabilitation is to occur. First, you do this by the realization that all of your attitudes, body language, behavior, and conversation influences the psychic energy of your patient. Next, all your conversation during physcial restoration treatments whether humorous, deeply philosophical, technically pragmatic, an exchange of knowledge, caring in nature, or seemingly casual has a lasting effect on the psychic energy, physical energy, and physical performance of the person you are attempting to assist to a greater level of rehabilitation. Also, the treatment milieu to which you expose your patients can either enhance or detract from their healthy psychic energy. If the environment is only filled with the implements of treatment from disease, the healthy psychic energy has little to stimulate it. The healthy psyche actively needs to relate to nature and artistic expressions for its energy.

And if your patient's rehabilitation ends suddenly in death, it nonetheless was still a meaningful experience for each moment gave expression to healthy psychic energy. Each moment had dignity. The dignity of an individual's suffering made evident through many kinds of psychic expressions thus radiating out to the family, friends, society, and the world. When dignity prevails civilization receives a most important gift—humaneness.

REFERENCES

1. Freud, Sigmund *The Major Works of Sigmund Freud.* Encyclopedia Britannica, Inc., 1952

2. Arieti, Silvano *The Intrapsyche Self—Feeling, Cognition, and Creativity in Health and Mental Illness.* New York: Basic Books, Inc., 1967.

3. Searles, Harold F. *The Nonhuman Environment.* International Universities Press, Inc., 1960

4. Frankl, Viktor E. *Man's Search for Meaning.* New York: Washington Square Press, Inc., 1963

Occupational Therapy as Part of a Pulmonary Rehabilitation Program

R. Lynette Walsh, MBAOT, SROT, OTR, MEd

ABSTRACT. In the City of Hope Medical Respiratory Care (MRC) program occupational therapy is a dynamic, integral part of the rehabilitation process. Three broad and varying aspects of occupational therapy are covered. These consist of upper extremity exercises using both an arm ergometer and gravity resistive exercises, relaxation and stress management training, and a multifaceted approach to activities of daily living (ADL) training. The ADL training is carried out in both individual and group sessions and includes techniques of work efficiency and motion economy, proper body mechanics, and proper breathing techniques during daily activities. The occupational therapist is a member of the MRC treatment team and would be unable to function effectively with these patients without the support and assistance of other members. The studies referred to in this paper validate this use of occupational therapy in a Pulmonary Rehabilitation Program.

The Medical Respiratory Care (MRC) program for persons with chronic respiratory disease was initiated at the City of Hope National Medical Center in 1972. The City of Hope is a referral medical and research center of 212 beds specializing in the care of catastrophic and debilitating illnesses of persons of all ages. Occupational therapy has been an integral part of the MRC program

---

Educated in England, R. Lynette Walsh is a member of the British Association of Occupational Therapists and holds state registration in the United Kingdom. Her Masters degree is from Salisbury State College, Salisbury, MD. She is currently staff occupational therapist, City of Hope National Medical Center, Duarte, CA.

The author wishes to acknowledge Brian Tiep, MD, the MRC Team, M. Szamet, OTR, and H. M. Brown, OTR, for assistance in preparing this paper.

This article appears jointly in *Occupational Therapy for the Energy Deficient Patient* (The Haworth Press, 1986), and *Occupational Therapy in Health Care*, Volume 3, Number 1 (Spring 1986).

65

for most of its existence, and consistently for the past seven years. patients in the program are part of a treatment team that includes physicians, nurses, occupational therapist, physical therapist, social worker, respiratory therapist, dietitian, pharmacist, discharge planning nurse and respiratory technicians. Team members spend varying amounts of time with patients and their families in both group and individual sessions to carry out comprehensive regimens suited to each patient's particular needs.

REFERRAL AND ADMISSION

A patient is referred to the City of Hope Department of Respiratory Diseases by his own community physician. He is then evaluated as an out-patient by the MRC physician, nurse and social worker to determine whether he is a suitable candidate for the MRC program. Conditions of acceptance into both the in-patient and subsequent out-patient parts of the program are explained to the patient and any family members who accompany him. These conditions include first, having been diagnosed as having chronic lung disease, especially the obstructive types (COPD),[1] confirmed by pulmonary function data. (Patients with lung cancer are not usually seen in this program at the hospital.) The next condition is a contract which the patient must sign on admission to the program in which he agrees to participate in the program to the best of his ability. Patients who are admitted must have the motivation necessary to carry them through a physically and psychologically demanding program. The contract includes statements of mutual expectations regarding both the patient's own goals in participating in the program and the treatment goals determined by team members. The patient also agrees to give up smoking on admission and to remain a non-smoker after discharge. Breach of contract may result in early discharge from the program.

INITIAL STAGES OF THE PROGRAM

The progam begins with a three week in-patient stay at the City of Hope as a 'planned' admission. However, prior to admission, in order to establish base-line information for planning, each patient has a complete physical work-up at the hospital including personal history, laboratory screening, chest X-rays, ECG, and pulmonary function studies, including arterial blood gases. Each patient also engages in an incremental exercise stress test, walking on a treadmill, during which ECG telemetry monitoring is used as well as ear oximetry to determine oxygen saturation levels at different levels of exercise demand. A physician supervises these tests after which he prepares instructions for the occupational and physical therapists to guide the patient's exercise management once he is hospitalized. Oxygen needs during activity will have also been determined. All evaluation and testing information is charted to be available to the team members for reference during subsequent treatment.

During the three week admission each patient participates in a daily schedule of activity and instruction sessions. All team members have scheduled sessions for both instruction and practice during the week. The daily schedule starts at approximately 8:30 or 9:00 a.m. and continues until 4:00 or 4:30 p.m. Sessions are usually 50 to 60 minutes each and are arranged so that activity and exercises are interspersed with instruction sessions, where the patient is sitting. The patient is encouraged to be responsible for following the schedule and being at sessions on time. Medical treatments are coordinated with the schedule as much as possible. Family members can participate with the patient at any time. On Saturdays and Sundays the patients are encouraged to practice the new techniques independently and on Saturdays they do have an upper extremity exercise group session supervised by an occupational therapist.

OCCUPATIONAL THERAPY PROGRAM

Evaluation

Before any treatment activity is begun a two stage evaluation is undertaken by the occupational therapist, beginning the day the patient is admitted. The first part consists of establishing a data base through interview. This is to determine the patient's current functional level in activities of daily living (ADL) including his self-care, activities in home management, vocational activities, if any, leisure activities, along with activity tolerances and ways of handling stress. Environmental information is particularly important to learn such as where and how the patient lives, in what kind of setting, with whom he lives and who assists him when needed. Any special limitations such as problems with vision, hearing, sleeping and possible claustrophobia are also determined. Most importantly, effort is made to learn about the patient's motivation, attitudes and goals.

The evaluation next turns to physical performance: measurements of upper extremity range of motion, grip strength and upper extremity muscle power and sensation. General occupational therapy goals and treatment plans are developed from this information even though more tests ensue.

The second part of the occupational therapy evaluation involves an incremental exercise test in which the patient operates an upper extremity bicycle ergometer followed, a day or so later, by an endurance exercise test.[2] (See Figure I.) Exercises requiring arm endurance are used in the occupational therapy program since a positive relationship has been shown between increased levels of upper extremity endurance and increased abilities in ADL and other activities that contribute to a patient's quality of life.[2,3,5]

The two ergometer tests (incremental and endurance) establish the baseline for a progressive endurance program of upper extremity exercise. Patients are assigned one session on the arm ergometer per day (of up to 20 minutes), four days a week while an in-patient, with ECG telemetry monitoring used during these exercises as needed. The need for monitoring has usually been predetermined by the physician during the pre-admission incremental stress test.

Arm Ergometry—As Evaluation and Exercise

For the arm ergometer incremental test,[2] the patient initially pedals in one minute intervals, with 5 watt increments added in each successive interval, until evidence of symptoms appear. The patient is positioned sitting in front of the arm ergometer so that his elbow is at approximately 90° flexion when at the bottom of the cycle stroke. The ergometer is placed close enough to the patient to avoid excessive forward thrusting of the patient's shoulders during the cycling motion. (See Figure II.) At the completion of the test, the total number of watts applied is multiplied by the number of minutes the patient pedaled to yield a watt-minutes workload[4] score. Pre and post exercise pulse and blood pressure readings are also taken and post exercise dyspnea level is determined. Dyspnea estimations are made by instructing the patient to count from one to fifteen (or to say his name and address), noting how many breaths he takes to complete the assignment. This is scored on a 4 level scale: level 2 took 2 breaths, level 3 took 3 or more breaths and level 4 means the patient

Figure I

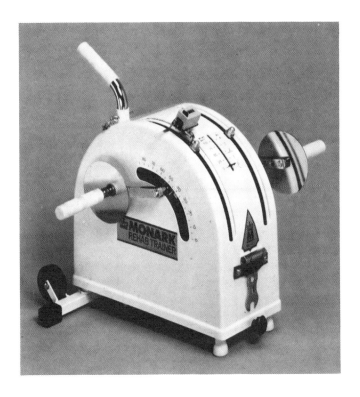

Arm Ergometer
Measurements: Length 540 mm. Width 470 mm.
Height 550 mm. Weight 21 kg.

can barely speak. This dyspnea information, repeatedly tested, is included in the patient's daily medical record and in weekly and discharge summaries.

During the next session using the arm ergometer (a day or so later) the patient is engaged in a test of sub-maximal arm endurance. For this he pedals against 50% of the maximum load achieved on the incremental test, for as long as possible, but to a maximum of 20 minutes. Pre and post exercise pulse and blood pressure readings are taken as before and post exercise dyspnea level is also determined. The watt-minutes workload in this test is calculated by

Figure II

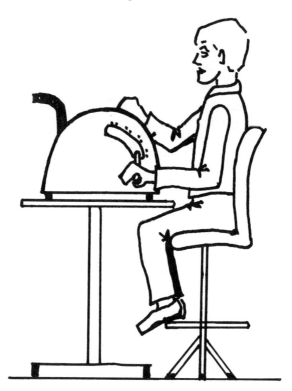

Patient positioning at the arm ergometer

multiplying the resistance applied by the number of minutes completed.

As the patient continues using arm ergometry four times a week, the number of minutes he was previously able to complete is increased 2-3 minutes per day, though keeping the same resistance level. Once the patient achieves a total of 20 minutes of exercise at the 50% base level, resistance is increased by 5 watts for the next session with the time period adjusted downwards to create a realistic workload goal for that session. The program would then stay at that now increased resistance level, gradually increasing the minutes completed over several sessions to a maximum of 20 minutes. In the next session the process would be repeated adding another 5 watts resistance and taking several sessions to work up to 20 minutes, and so on. Prior to discharge, a comparison is made between the workloads the patient was able to achieve on the initial incremental and endurance tests and the workload he has achieved in his last session. This usually shows quite dramatic gains and is most encouraging to the patient. An example would be B.L. who started at 140 watt-minutes workload and progressed to a workload of 450 watt-minutes prior to discharge. His shortness of breath decreased from a level 3 to a level 1, even with the higher workload. Subjectively patients report less shortness of breath and less difficulty with activities where their arms are elevated (for example shampoo) or loaded (for example lifting and carrying things) as well as the positive relationship between these exercises and improved ADL performance shown in our study.[5]

Other Exercise Activities

In addition to using upper extremity ergometer exercises, the occupational therapist instructs a patient in a series of gravity resistive exercises for the upper extremity that become part of his exercise 'prescription' for a home program. In order to set the stage for success in home carry-over all patients are given responsibility for doing the exercises during their hospitalization. They demonstrate this responsibility initially by learning the movements, understanding the reasons for them and then doing the exercises correctly while supervised by the occupational therapist. They are encouraged to establish a routine for doing the exercises regularly while still in the hospital in order to be ready to continue this same routine after discharge. On admission each patient receives a notebook in which to accumulate information about every aspect of the program, including his progress for future reference. Patients accumulate notes from teaching sessions as well as hand-out materials from classes and other sessions with staff. The notebook becomes a major resource. In it are included exercise routines as well as their own 'scores' on various tests to chart their progress.

Relaxation and Stress Management

Relaxation and stress management are important components of the COPD program content in occupational therapy. The rationale for including relaxation and stress management training is that program history shows that a great majority of patients who have been seen complain of increased shortness of breath when stressed and anxious. Also approximately 50% of the patients describe types of claustrophobia and 'panic' attacks associated with extreme tension and shortness of breath. Therefore, specific strategies to address these needs have been developed.

The occupational therapist provides group sessions in relaxation training for patients three times a week during their three week stay. Following the philosophies of the Bernstein and Borkovec method of progressive relaxation training,[6] three out of a possible six 'scripts' have been developed for use with the MRC patients. The script involves the occupational therapist instructing the patients in a systematic method of tensing and relaxing specific muscle groups. Usually the arms are done first, then the head and neck, shoulders, back, chest, and abdomen and lastly the legs and feet. The patients are supine in a quiet, semi-dark room for best results. Two of the scripts involve tension release and the third is a progression to recall where the patient is able to relax without actually tensing the muscles first.

This progressive method is used so that both patients with experience in relaxation and those who have never been exposed to relaxation techniques can learn suitable strategies easily without added stress. The variety of approaches available in the scripts also serves the different needs patients will have as they apply the techniques in their own life patterns and life styles later. The techniques are presented to patients with the intent that they incorporate them as part of their daily routines as well as to assist with sleeping, and, in emergency use, for panic control. Each patient is also provided with a cassette tape of the training sessions so that he has a ready reference and support to use while in the hospital if needed, and later as part of his home program after discharge. This has proven effective as a way of supporting patients in developing habits of relaxation and stress reduction.

Training in assertiveness is also part of the stress management program taught by the occupational therapist. Initially discussions with patients explain the differences between assertive, aggressive and passive behaviors. Then role playing is used to illustrate these behaviors and to offer ways for patients to demonstrate and practice specific assertive techniques. Situations critical to a patient with COPD are used. Such things as how does one ask someone not to smoke, ask a relative or friend not to use certain cologne or per-

fume, or how can one negotiate a change of roles and responsibilities in the household to accommodate one's own energy levels.
Learning techniques such as these enables a patient to have control
over stressful situations, empowers him to do something construc-
tive about solving problems, and offers ways to enhance his self-
esteem in the process. Patients welcome such new skills and are
greatly helped by learning to use them. Also the group process lends
much support to such behavioral changes.

ADL Related Activities

In addition to the exercise and stress management programs, and
closely related to them, patients engage with the occupational therapist in both individual and group sessions in order to learn and try
information and activity, and relate these to improved function in
daily activities. For this aspect of the program group training sessions are scheduled for one hour twice a week when basic factual information is given, supported by written hand-outs, audio-visual
aids and actual practice activities. During practice sessions patients
are encouraged to demonstrate the techniques they have just
learned, giving support and encouragement to one another and even
critique, as needed.

The major topics in this part of the occupational therapy program
are given in rotation so that each patient is exposed to all of them in
his three week stay. They include techniques of work efficiency and
motion economy, proper body mechanics and proper breathing
techniques during daily activities. The activities especially empha-
sized are self care, including use of adaptive equipment, household
chores, kitchen activities, marketing, bed-making and the hazards
of products used in ADL (e.g., cleaners, polishes, sprays, etc.).
Energy costs as critical variables in activity choice and ways of performing the activity are discussed and incorporated into time management techniques applicable to each patient's own lifestyle.

Classes are structured to enable patients to be active participants
in the sessions and also to demonstrate a self-help philosophy by
sharing both their own experiences and their ways of solving ADL
problems. Observation and discussion are key strategies used during
practice sessions to insure that each patient is learning and applying
techniques correctly. All team members support patients in becoming independent self-starters in using their learned exercise and
other routines outside class time and ultimately at home. When

problems arise in any aspect of the MRC program they are discussed either individually by one team member or in a patient/team conference. In occupational therapy, family members are especially encouraged to participate in both instruction sessions and conferences so that they can understand the program and support the patient's participation in it. Team members also try to share with each other information they use in teaching/counseling to promote consistency when information is communicated to the patient and family.

Individually monitored evaluations of self-care activities are done by the occupational therapist on an as-needed basis. Bathing, drying off, dressing and hair care are the activities usually observed during such an evaluation, with ECG telemetry monitoring used if indicated. In keeping with class information, patients are encouraged to practice pacing themselves and working on breathing control during activities. If a patient requires continuous oxygen, this is used during activity and he is taught how to use it appropriately, as physician prescribed.

Team Conferences and Rounds

Team conferences and regular communication among staff members of the MRC team are critical elements in the success of a program in which patients are being helped to make significant life style changes. As a member of the MRC team, the occupational therapist attends two formal team sessions each week. One conference, with each member reporting progress, is essentially a planning meeting. The other includes the patient and if possible his family members, since patient and family understanding and cooperation is fundamental to program success. Throughout the three week patient stay, in all contacts with staff, patients are encouraged to participate in following their progress and in understanding what the objective information from repeated exercises and tests means. After daily sessions, for example, they are given vital sign and workload information and they record this in their notebooks. Then when in the conference each team member summarizes the patient's progress in that aspect of his progam, the patient can better understand the information. If a patient is having difficulty with any aspect of his program, the time of the conference is when this can be discussed and strategies negotiated for resolving the problem.

EFFECTIVENESS OF THE
OCCUPATIONAL THERAPY PROGRAM

Both subjective and objective information has been examined in determining the effectiveness of both the rationale and strategies of occupational therapy in this rehabilitation program for patients with COPD. In an occupational therapy quality assurance study done in 1983,[7] a 26% improvement over a three week period was recorded in the patients' retention and use of knowledge of ADL work efficiency techniques, in proper breathing patterns during ADL, in use of adaptive equipment for energy conservation during ADL, in use of relaxation and stress management techniques and upper extremity exercises. This improvement was based on changes noted between data collected from the patients on admission to the three week program and then on discharge.

Another study compared scores of subjective symptoms and objective data.[5] A positive relationship was shown between increased upper extremity endurance and increased ability to perform daily living activities. In objective data from arm ergometer exercises, the mean upper extremity endurance for a group of 23 patients improved from 166 to 372 watt-minutes workload. This was accompanied by a significant decrease in difficulty with ADL. The ADL information was based on each patient rating himself on an activity scale. Data were collected on admission, at discharge and six months after discharge when an out-patient. From discharge to six months post, the subjective gains remained the same.

In another study, in comparing activity levels and self care ability over the period of a year, ADL ability improved between admission and discharge, and was maintained at six months and a year, with no significant reduction for either men or women.[8] When the data on admission were compared with data at one year, the improvement had dropped slightly for both men and the combined group. But there was a significant increase in the ability for women. The conclusion is that since both objective and subjective symptom measures of endurance and ADL improved, it appears that this approach to rehabilitation can exert a practical lasting effect on patients with COPD.

Subjective feedback from patients indicate good results and enjoyment, especially from the relaxation and stress management training sessions. Outpatients on return visits indicated further that they continued to use the techniques at home. Studies involving both objective and subjective data are being planned to validate the techniques for relaxation and stress management used in occupational therapy.

The MRC team has also used compliance[9] as an indicator of the value and lasting effect of the rehabilitation methods used in this program. During occupational therapy, as noted previously, the patients are instructed in a series of gravity resistive exercises for the upper extremities. These exercises then become part of the patient's home program. As part of the out-patient follow-up, patients have regularly scheduled clinic visits over 6-12 months depending on the patient's circumstances and proximity to the hospital. Compliance information from such visits was erratic and purely subjective. Therefore, to substantiate and improve compliance, a weekly out-patient group was begun.[9] Specific data are collected from each patient to determine his progress, including the effects of the upper extremity exercises taught to him by the occupational therapist. Over a period of three years, it was found that 74% of the patient population was complying with the exercise routines on the first visit (after discharge from the three week in-patient portion of the program); 19% had not complied; and 7% had medical reasons for non-compliance. On the second return to the group, compliance improved to 88%; and non-compliance dropped to 12%. These data were based on 212 patients and a total of 455 visits to the 'compliance' group. During these group sessions, not only are performance data collected from each patient, but also counseling and encouragement by team members and the peer group of other MRC graduates occurs to help participants comply with exercise prescriptions. Team members also lend support and answer questions that arise. The positive encouragement and support that result are key elements to compliance.

CONCLUSIONS

Although this occupational therapy program covers a wide spectrum of occupational therapy techniques, its effectiveness can be seen in patient performance as well as in documented studies. This is especially noticeable when looking at the way exercise facilitates the patient's ability to increase function and is not an end in itself. Subjective responses from patients also support this. This program continues as described but is always subject to review and change in order to meet the patients' needs. One of the exciting challenges of the program is being able to validate outcomes and patient responses, to develop new techniques, and confirm established ones without losing the fun and humanity of working with this patient population.

SUMMARY

In the City of Hope Medical Respiratory Care program, occupational therapists cover three broad treatment areas: prescriptive upper extremity exercise, a varied ADL program which incorporates principles of energy conservation and efficient body use, and relaxation and stress management training. All parts of the program are directed toward helping patients to understand their energy levels and activity potentials and to increase their abilities to engage successfully in the activities of daily living of their chosen life style. The program is stuctured in a way that respects each patient as an individual and helps him realize his potential as a functioning member of his family and of society. Several studies are reported which validate the types of strategies used in implementing the occupational therapy program. Occupational therapy is definitely significant in helping patients to resume meaningful and productive lives.

REFERENCES

1. Tiep, B: Intensive approach to pulmonary rehabilitation. *City of Hope Quarterly* 8:6-9, 1979

2. Butts, J: Pulmonary rehabilitation through exercise and education. *CVP* Dec/Jan 1981

3. Belman, M J: Exercise physiology and its application in the training of patients with COPD. *City of Hope Quarterly* 8:3-5 1979

4. Astrand P O, Rodahl, K: *Textbook of Work Physiology.* New York: McGraw Hill Book Co., 1970, 1977

5. Anderson, L K, Tiep, B, Belman, M J, Walsh, R L, Butts, J R: Objective & Subjective Improvement After Exercise Training in Patients With COPD. American Thoracic Society, April 1983

6. Bernstein, D A, Borkovec, T D: Progressive Relaxation Training—A Manual for the Helping Professions. Champaign, Illnois: Research Press, 1973

7. Walsh, R L, Szamet, M: Occupational Therapy Quality Assurance Study. City of Hope Rehabilitation Department, June 1983. Unpublished study

8. Anderson, L K, Tiep, B L, Belman, M J, Walsh, R L, Lewis, Y: Results of One Year Follow up After Pulmonary Rehabilitation in Patients With COPD. American Thoracic Society. December 1984

9. Walsh, R L: Out-Patient Compliance With Occupational Therapy Exercises for Patients With COPD. City of Hope Rehabilitation Department. March 1985. Unpublished study

A Subjective ADL Rating Scale for the Pulmonary Rehabilitation Patient

Margaret A. Phillips, MS, OTR

ABSTRACT. A subjective rating scale to measure changes in performance of activities of daily living before and after participation in an out-patient multidisciplinary pulmonary rehabilitation program is presented. Results of a small pilot study using the scale is reported in which the scores of patients in ADL are compared with one measure of their pulmonary function. The use of the scale as an adjunct to planning occupational therapy programs is proposed and suggestions are made both for its change and for improving its usefulness to other therapists.

Outpatients in the Pulmonary Rehabilitation Program at San Jose Hospital (SJH) participate in a program that offers a team approach to treatment. Services consist of occupational therapy for energy conservation, relaxation techniques, task analysis and learning to coordinate breathing patterns with activity demands; physical therapy for exercise and conditioning; respiratory therapy for evaluation of the nature and severity of the respiratory disease, breathing instruction and education about lung conditions. In addition, a dietitian and social worker may work with patients individually or in groups. Those in each discipline are responsible for developing and using measurement devices to establish bases for treatment and to check for changes in behavior and performance noted during the

Margaret A. Phillips has directed the occupational therapy services at San Jose Hospital, San Jose, CA, since 1972. She has both a BS and MS in occupational therapy from San Jose State University.

The author wishes to thank Sidney Choslovsky, MD, Medical Director of the Pulmonary Rehabilitation Program, and Carol Wienecke, RRT, Supervisor, Respiratory Therapy, for their assistance in manuscript preparation.

This article appears jointly in *Occupational Therapy for the Energy Deficient Patient* (The Haworth Press, 1986) and *Occupational Therapy in Health Care,* Volume 3, Number 1 (Spring 1986).

79

length of the program. The occupational therapy staff have developed a subjective activities of daily living (ADL) rating scale to be completed by patients as part of their initial evaluation, at discharge, and again at recheck intervals. This paper will briefly describe the scale and its use in a small pilot study in which attempts were made to both identify patient needs, their changes as result of the program and how performance correlated with levels of pulmonary function as measure by the $FEV_{1.0}$ (forced expiratory volume in one second) test.

The use of a subjective rating in pulmonary rehabilitation has been suggested as an aid to goal setting by both patient and therapist. Hodgkin[1,p80] urged that goals be set from 'a previously measured or subjectively experienced baseline.' In-patient programs offer opportunity to work with patients in self care and other tasks that are not feasible within the time frames of outpatient programs. In the SJH out-patient program patients are scheduled for two hour blocks of time for treatment by the team, twice weekly. The occupational therapy portion of the four hour weekly period is accomplished in 30 to 60 minute sessions, and any one patient is usually seen for no more than a total of ten hours by occupational therapy during an outpatient regimen. Within these constraints the use of a subjective rating scale was seen as helpful for planning programs that would be effective and efficient.

THE RATING SCALE

The SJH rating scale was developed and refined to its present state by the occupational therapy staff rotating through the Pulmonary Rehabilitation Service at the hospital. In it three levels of performance are considered, with sub-categories within each level. See Figure I. In the first level are listed personal *Self Care* tasks such as eating, dressing, hygiene, and grooming. The activities in the second level, *Household,* require greater work tolerance levels because they combine standing, walking, use of arms, bending, reaching, lifting, carrying—all higher energy demand activities. Such tasks as meal preparation, vacuuming, sweeping are included as typical daily tasks. In the third level, *Outdoors,* activities that are still more demanding are listed. In general they require not only the energy/effort of self-care and household tasks but also a high degree of work tolerance or endurance. Included are such activities as going on a community outing, shopping, attending church, traveling.

The scale is introduced and completed by the patient during an initial evaluation, again at discharge and again when he is seen during return recheck visits. The original test form is purposely used again at retest (note the rating columns, Figure I) so that the patient is able to compare initial, discharge and/or recheck scores by referring to his previous scorings. Seeing one's previous scores is considered important due to the need for realistic goal setting. In order

SAN JOSE HOSPITAL
OCCUPATIONAL THERAPY

SUBJECTIVE ADL RATING SCALE FOR THE PULMONARY REHABILITATION PATIENT

Name: _____ Age: _____ Date: _____

Your doctor has ordered occupational therapy for you. This is a service which can teach you how to save energy and show you how to conserve your breath when doing simple living tasks. The therapist would like to know what areas cause you to be overly tired, short of breath, or most distressed.

Indicate how well you perform these tasks. Use numbers 1-10, with 10 being the highest or best possible ease of accomplishing the task and 5 being with difficulty or shortness of breath, even if the difficulty is only at times and you recover quickly. Use 1-2 if you no longer do the task or must have it done for you. Use numbers between 1,5,10, to indicate levels of difficulty that fall between these major levels.

Filling out this check list will act as a guideline for you and the therapist to work from. Please think the questions over and answer them carefully.

Indicate how you perform these tasks:	Initial	At Discharge	At Recheck
A. Self Care			
1. Dressing			
a. shirt			
b. pants			
c. shoes/socks			
2. Shaving/washing face			
3. Combing your hair			
4. Bathing: tub/shower			
5. Toweling off			
B. Household Chores			
1. Getting from room to room			
2. Simple Repairs			
3. Making simple foods(coffee, toast, etc.)			
4. Preparing a meal			
5. Taking out the trash			
6. Cleaning			
a. washing dishes			
b. dusting			
c. vacuuming			
d. washing clothes			
e. sinks/bathtubs			
C. Out Doors			
1. Driving			
2. Shopping			
3. Gardening			
4. Attending events(sports,movies,etc.)			
5. Visiting			
6. Traveling			
7. Hobbies			

Figure I

to get overall function scores, the therapist totals the ratings. This is done within each level first, dividing the total score by the number of items marked, thus getting a final subscore for each level of tasks: Self Care, Household, and Outdoors.

Instructions for scoring are printed above the rating scale itself, and patients are asked to read the instructions prior to filling out the scale. Therapists make certain they understand the process by giving examples of ratings. In the study to be reported, one therapist administered all of the evaluations and her presentations were made as similar as possible from patient to patient. The examples of levels of scoring explained by the therapist—the highest score possible (10), a middle score (5), helped patients to understand the purpose of the ratings as well as clarified any questions they had prior to rating themselves.

A PILOT STUDY

A six month pilot study using the scale was designed to use both the total scores and those on individual items specifically in helping patients to set goals for their program and to guide therapists in programming. Scores were also later used to compare ADL function with scores on one pulmonary function test. Even though the study has concluded, the scale is still being used and gradually modified to reflect changes deemed necessary from its use in the study.

Twenty patients completed the initial scale, fifteen patients completed the discharge rating. Five of the original were prematurely discharged from the program due to medical complications so the data from their initial scores have not been included in the study. In addition, five of the original group completed all parts of the process in the study but because of incomplete pulmonary function data have also been excluded from tabulations. Therefore, final N is 10, admittedly small, but seen as enough to get a beginning feel for the usefulness of the instrument. Patients included represented diagnoses of emphysema, chronic bronchitis, chronic obstructive pulmonary disease (COPD), and in the cases of two subjects, accompanying asthma.

While usual pulmonary function tests consist of several subtests, for the study only the forced expiratory volume in one second ($FEV_{1.0}$) was selected. This is because it is a measurement widely used and understood by professionals working with respiratory patients. The $FEV_{1.0}$ value is often used as a general indicator of prognosis as well. Changes appear in the $FEV_{1.0}$ values before a patient complains of dyspnea.[1,p18] Therefore it was hypothesized that persons who scored themselves high on the subjective scale would still demonstrate lower than normal $FEV_{1.0}$ values consistent with their respiratory diagnosis indicating either that they had not carefully considered how activities affected them, or that they had not recognized their disability. Therefore the program might not produce significant change in their scores. On the other hand, it was felt that persons who gave themselves low scores on a subjective scale would probably evidence more dyspnea symptoms and correspondingly lower $FEV_{1.0}$ values since they apparently knew they had problems. Correspondingly they would have potential for improving performance from programming.

RESULTS OF THE STUDY

Staff had expected to see initial scores averaging 6-7, indicating shortness of breath, in Self Care tasks, and slightly lower scores, averaging 5-6, in the more demanding Household and Outdoor tasks. A rise in these initial scores was anticipated at the end of the program. Instead, half of the persons in the study demonstrated little or no change in initial versus discharge scores. These became Group A. The other half, who tended to support the predictions became Group B. They were the persons whose scores fell into predicted averages (based on diagnosis, age and sex) and showed a rise (improvement) in scores at discharge. The $FEV_{1.0}$ values for each group were then averaged to compare with ADL averages in each grading period. See Figure II.

Figure II

Average Scores for ADL Sub-categories

Group	$FEV_{1.0}$		Self Care	Household	Outdoor
A	39%	initial	8.4	7.4	6.8
		discharge	8.7	8.0	7.1
B	28%	initial	5.9	4.3	3.8
		discharge	7.2	5.5	5.9

Group A

The patients in Group A (N = 5) had average initial scores of 8.4 for Self Care, 7.4 for Household and 6.8 for Outdoor tasks. At the same time the average $FEV_{1.0}$ value was 39% of predicted normal values (normal and acceptable being 70-100%). At the end of the program, the average scores in Self Care had increased to 8.7, in Household to 8.0 and in Outdoor, to 7.1. A short case study will illustrate those typical of Group A.

Case I

Mr. L, a retired 67 year old man, entered the Pulmonary Rehabilitation Program two weeks after a newly diagnosed COPD condition which he had first noticed while on vacation when he was unable to work on his motorhome while parked at a high elevation. He scored himself on all Self Care tasks in the 9 levels with an average score of 9, Household tasks in the 8,9,10 levels, averaging 8.6 and Outdoor tasks as 1,3,9,10 levels with an average of 5.9. While the patient claimed at discharge that he had improved because of the program, his scores remained essentially unchanged. Self Care scores actually lowered to an average of 8.7, Household scores remained at 8.6, and Outdoor scores raised slightly to 6.1. His $FEV_{1.0}$ value was at 67% of predicted normal.

Mr. L's case from Group A well illustrates one problem with using the subjective rating scale, that persons may give themselves high initial scores if newly diagnosed and in relatively good health otherwise. Mr. L had suffered an acute onset which he initially feared was cardiac in nature, had been surprised by the diagnosis and had had little time to correlate his gradual decline in activity performance with a medical condition. His $FEV_{1.0}$ value was one of the highest in the study (almost in normal ranges) and therefore he was the least impaired person in Group A. He denied having experienced dyspnea in Self Care activities as evidenced by his subjective rating scale scores. He was, however, able to examine a specific task or activity, learn to analyze and correct breathing patterns during a task and therefore recognize significant improvements in his lifestyle as a result of the occupational therapy intervention. The energy conservation and task analysis components of the program proved helpful to him in reducing fatigue and discomfort in performing tasks. Even though he was able to recognize improvements in his performance, however, he still graded himself at discharge slightly lower in Self Care, retained the same scores in Household and raised them slightly in Outdoor tasks. he concluded that his estimates of his performance initially must have been too high and that those scores should have been lower. His conversations suggested that he was accepting the COPD condition but until the end of the program he still had little awareness of how it affected his lifestyle. The gradual onset had contributed to a slow decline in function which the patient had associated with 'the aging process.' Once diagnosed and instructed in pulmonary rehabilitation strategies, Mr. L recognized he indeed had achieved a higher level of function.

In essence there may always be a problem in using the subjective scale with newly diagnosed persons or with those who have not been able to relate their diminished function to pulmonary disease. Nonetheless, the scale can still form a good basis for education and counseling with patients to help them to focus on how their own awareness of performance can influence the scope and range of activities they want to do.

Group B

The patients in Group B (N = 5) produced scores that are more like those staff had expected for their ages and diagnoses. They proved to be persons who had had definitive problems in doing activity before using the rating scale (dyspnea on activity) and thus their scores reflected recognition of problems. Group B patients showed initial scores averaging 5.9 in Self Care, 4.3 in Household and 3.8 in Outdoor tasks, quite low in contrast to those in Group A. Discharge scores averaged 7.2 in Self Care, 5.5 in Household and 5.9 in Outdoor tasks. Also, their $FEV_{1.0}$ values averaged only 28% of predicted normal, some 11% lower than Group A. Based upon these scores and conversations with individuals, the persons in this group tended to confirm an initial awareness of breathing problems (and an openness to help to improve their function) and did each show improvement by the end of the program in their level of performance.

In this group, despite instruction in scoring, patients rated themselves no lower than 4 if they continued to perform a given task, even though they did so with extreme difficulty. In light of their lower $FEV_{1.0}$ values one could well have anticipated even lower self-rating scores on the scales. Mrs. T's case will illustrate Group B persons who typically reported dyspnea during self care tasks and rated themselves as improved, with less dyspnea, during tasks at discharge.

Case II

Mrs. T is a 52 year old woman with a short history of breathing problems and an acute onset of respiratory distress one month preceding referral to the program. She rated herself initially with scores from low to moderate levels. She had been vacationing and experienced severe respiratory distress requiring hospitalization. She scored herself at 6.8 for Self Care tasks, but for Household tasks and Outdoor tasks dropped to 6.1 and 4.0 respectively. She was fearful of activity because of her shortness of breath and said her goal was simply to be able to resume her role as a housewife. After engaging in the rehabilitation regimen in occupational therapy, her scores at discharge rose considerably, averaging 8.6 for Self Care, 7.5 for Household and 5.3 for Outdoor tasks. While her $FEV_{1.0}$ was only 15% of predicted normal, a highly impaired pulmonary function score, and the lowest of any of the Group B participants, it is surprising that she rated herself as high as she did.

Mrs. T obviously had an awareness of her condition and its effects on her daily routines. While at discharge the severity of her condition was still not fully understood by her, the contrast between her initial and discharge scores, as well as her conversation with staff and other patients, revealed a better degree of acceptance and understanding of her limitations. She also showed an ability to apply the principles presented in the program in practical and functional ways. At discharge she described herself as being able to pace herself better to plan for a day of activity matching her energy levels and to demonstrate better tolerance for the work planned. Also having learned how to coordinate her breathing with Self Care and Household tasks, she was honestly able to score her performance of daily activities higher at discharge.

SUMMARY AND CONCLUSIONS

A subjective self-rated activities of daily living scale was developed and used in a pilot study with pulmonary rehabilitation outpatients at San Jose Hospital as a pre and post test to explore how patients perceive the limitations of pulmonary disease. It was intended to assist the occupational therapist in measuring behavior in activities of daily living and to plan instruction and counseling in energy conservation, relaxation techniques, ways of coordinating breathing with activity and how one can analyze tasks so as to perform them without or with less stress. It would also help indicate results of programming.

When the scores of the small pilot group were studied, they revealed that patients tended to fall into two groups based both on levels of their intial scores and by amounts of change noted at discharge. Those results have been described and discussed through use of two cases. Since the scoring did divide the test group into two rather distinct groups, it may have value not only to guide planning of education/program for patients but also to give clearer indications for evaluating newly diagnosed persons, those who may not yet have absorbed the full implications of pulmonary disease.

However, individual scoring in both groups seemed to require a more discrete scale for indicating levels of difficulty. Adjustments of both activities included, instructions to patients and the scales themselves are planned for further study. Also while it is seen as important to relate scores to $FEV_{1.0}$ values, additional data will be needed to see how well the scales discriminate levels of difficulty in daily activity as expected from their $FEV_{1.0}$ values.

It is felt that a subjective rating scale can be useful in an outpatient Pulmonary Rehabilitation Program not only in identifying patient problems in ADL performance but also in measuring changes in performance after being taught by the occupational therapist. If a scale can give patients practical perceptions of the effects of their pulmonary disease it would seem to follow that their interest in and responses to program would be enhanced. Only further development and use of the SJH scale will begin to confirm those assumptions. Other occupational therapists in pulmonary programs are invited to develop and/or share similar attempts at quantifying entry and discharge levels of patient performance or to make suggestions for the improvement of the one reported.

REFERENCES

1. Hodgkin, JE, ed., *Chronic obstructive pulmonary disease: Current concepts in diagnosis and comprehensive care.* Park Ridge, IL: American College of Chest Physicians, 1979, p80, 18

SUGGESTED READINGS

1. Bebout, DE, et al.: Clinical and physiological outcomes of a university-hospital pulmonary rehabilitation program. *Resp Care,* 28: 1468-1473, 1983

2. Berzina, GF: An occupational therapy program for the chronic obstructive pulmonary disease patient. *Am J Occup Ther* 24: 181-186, 1970

3. Cherniack, RM: *Pulmonary Function Testing,* Philadelphia: W.B. Saunders Co, 1977

4. Hodgkin, JE, ed: *Pulmonary Rehabilitation: Guidelines to Success,* Stoneham, MA: Butterworth Publishers, 1984

5. MacDonell, RJ: Suggestions for establishment of pulmonary rehabilitation programs. *Resp Care* 26, 966-977, 1981

6. Nicol, J, et al.: Strategies for developing a cost-effective pulmonary rehabilitation program. *Resp Care* 28:1451-1455,1983

7. Petty, TL: Pulmonary rehabilitation—better living with new techniques. *Resp Care* 30:98-107,1985

8. Pomerantz et al.: Occupational therapy for chronic obstructive lung disease. *Am J Occup Ther* 29:407-411,1975

9. Wright, RW, et al.: Benefits of a community-hospital pulmonary rehabilitation program. *Resp Care* 28:1474-1479,1983

Monitored Dressing Evaluation: Physiologic Assessment of Cardiac Work Tolerance

Eleanor Haid, OTR

ABSTRACT. The ability to measure changes in self care status for patients with cardiovascular disease is difficult to quantify since their independence is not usually limited by the need for physical assistance. Instead, limitations may include changes in vital signs that indicate excessive workload for the cardiovascular system, abnormally slow work pace, or inability to perform other tasks due to fatigue after self care is completed. Typical parameters that have been used to measure improvement in work tolerance, such as the ability to work for longer periods of time at progressively higher workloads, do not apply to self care.

The purpose of this paper is to describe a monitored dressing evaluation that includes a scale to grade functional work tolerance. The scoring system provides a more objective way than usually available to measure improvements in tolerance for dressing. It is especially useful for the patient at a low level of function.

Occupational therapists have monitored the work tolerance of patients with diminished cardiac reserve since the 1950's.[1,2,3] The use of graded activity programs by occupational therapists to increase the work tolerance of cardiac convalescents paralleled advances in cardiac rehabilitation and early mobilization of patients post-myocardial infarction. In these programs, occupational therapists assessed the work tolerance of their patients by using known

Eleanor Haid is Supervisor of Occupational Therapy on the cardiac unit at The Burke Rehabilitation Center in White Plains, NY.

The author would like to gratefully acknowledge Ronnie Schein, OTR, and the occupational therapists on the cardiac team at Burke for their assistnce in developing the scoring system for the functional work tolerance scale.

This article appears jointly in *Occupational Therapy for the Energy Deficient Patient* (The Haworth Press, 1986) and *Occupational Therapy in Health Care,* Volume 3, Number 1 (Spring 1986).

energy cost tables, and by physiologic monitoring. Heart rate and symptoms were monitored before, during, and after activities, using specific physiological response guidelines. A patient's progress could then be measured by performance of activities at a higher energy demand, ability to work at a particular energy demand for longer periods of time, changes in heart rate (HR) responses to activities, or reduction in symptoms.

More recently, occupational therapists have added monitoring of blood pressure (BP), auscultation of heart sounds, and radiotelemetry EKG monitoring to HR and symptom monitoring in their assessment of work tolerance. Specific guidelines are used for progression of self care, homemaking, vocational, and avocational activity programs, as well as exercise programs.[4,5,6,7]

Being able to monitor self care status is of particular interest to therapists since most cardiac patients routinely perform self care when in the subacute phase. Although dressing and grooming are commonly listed as low energy demand tasks on various energy cost charts,[7,8] it has been noted that there is wide variability in HR and BP responses to self care tasks among individuals independent of the energy cost of the activity. HR and BP responses are significant because they indicate the actual workload of the heart. Although some patients may be working at a low percentage of their maximal capacity while doing self care, others may be working at levels close to their maximum capacity. In monitored self care evaluation of 120 patients, post-myocardial infarction, Ogden found considerable variation in HR response to self care.[4] The distribution of maximal HR was unrelated to the known energy demand of the activity. Monitored self care evaluations are used to establish safe guidelines for independent resumption of self care and as a tool for instruction in energy saving techniques.

Monitored self care evaluations can also be used to measure changes in a patient's functional work tolerance for self care activities. It may be difficult to quantify improvements in self care status in patients with cardiac disease, since most of them are able to complete such tasks without physical assistance. Limiting factors tend to be significant changes in vital signs that indicate excessive cardiac workload, slow work pace, or symptoms such as shortness of breath, fatigue or chest pain. These factors are difficult to quantify in order to demonstrate improvement. Other parameters that have been used to document improvements in work tolerance for cardiac patients, such as the ability to work for increasingly longer periods of time at progressively higher workloads, are not appropriate for activities such as getting dressed since dressing is usually performed in a short amount of time at a relatively constant workload. Therefore, a different method must be used to measure progress.

One way of noting changes in self care status is to use a system that classifies a patient's functional work tolerance in terms of good, fair, or poor. Progress is noted as the patient's work tolerance changes from one grade to another. Factors that contribute to functional work tolerance for self care include:

1. HR and BP responses
2. the length of time required to complete the activity
3. the number of rest periods during the activity
4. the severity of symptoms
5. the amount of recovery time required upon completion of the activity.

The functional work tolerance grade can be added to the monitored self care evaluation to provide information for documentation of changes in status.

Figure 1 illustrates a monitored dressing evaluation that is used at the Burke Rehabilitation Center in White Plains, NY. It was designed to be used with adult patients with cardiac disease who are deconditioned or who have severe permanent impairments in cardiovascular and/or pulmonary function. It is also used with complicated or high risk cardiac patients who are monitored more closely and progressed at a slower rate than uncomplicated patients or those with mild impairments. The evaluation is done upon admission to the rehabilitation center, usually between 10 days and 4 weeks after myocardial infarction (MI) or cardiac surgery. Although it was designed for cardiac patients, it may be used for pulmonary patients or other types of patients who have low endurance. Use of the evaluation with these patients would require some modifications of the rating scale.

THE EVALUATION PROCESS

HR may be monitored by palpation of pulse, by auscultation using a stethoscope, by pulse meters, or by radiotelemetry EKG monitoring. Auscultation and radiotelemetry monitoring are more accurate than pulse palpation to obtain the HR. Radiotelemetry monitoring also provides information about heart rhythm and ischemic changes.

Figure 1

BURKE REHABILITATION CENTER

OCCUPATIONAL THERAPY DEPARTMENT MONITORED DRESSING EVALUATION

NAME: _____ DIAGNOSIS: _____ AGE: ____ DATE: _____

A. STATUS: UE _____ LE _____ SOCKS _____ SHOES _____

Comment: _____

Equipment/Adaptations: _____

B. VITAL SIGNS

	HEART RATE	BLOOD PRESSURE R or L	RESPIRATIONS
BEFORE seated ‑‑‑‑‑‑‑‑‑‑ standing			
AFTER			
2 MINUTES			
5 MINUTES			

C. TIME: _____   D. NUMBER OF REST PERIODS _____

E. SYMPTOMS: Fatigue _____ Shortness of Breath _____ Angina _____

Dizziness (when) _____ Pain (where) _____

Other: _____

F. BORG RATING: _____

G. INCORPORATION OF LABOR SAVING TECHNIQUES:

Spontaneous _____ Cues _____ N/A or Unable _____

H. INCORPORATION OF BREATHING TECHNIQUES (if applicable):

Spontaneous _____ Cues _____ N/A or Unable _____

I. VALSALVA ON EXERTION: No ____ Yes ____ N/A or not observed ____

J. FUNCTIONAL WORK TOLERANCE: Good ____ Fair ____ Poor ____

Expensive equipment is not necessary, however, to perform a monitored dressing evaluation. It may be done with a stethoscope, a blood pressure cuff, and a watch or clock with a second hand. The components of the evaluation follow.

THE EVALUATION COMPONENTS

A. STATUS: The amount of physical assistance required is noted. Common categories include: Independent, Observation, Minimal-Moderate-Maximal Assistance, or Dependent. Note if cues are required or if adaptive devices are used.

B. VITAL SIGNS: Techniques for monitoring HR and BP have been reported by Ogden[9,10] and Shanfield.[11] HR, BP, and respirations are monitored, in that order, prior to dressing, immediately upon completion, and after 2 minutes of seated rest. Readings are repeated at 5 minutes if pre-activity levels are not reached at 2 minutes. They can be repeated at 5 minute intervals thereafter until readings return to pre-activity levels. Peak HR should be checked during difficult aspects of dressing, and all readings should be taken whenever the patient experiences moderate to severe symptoms. All readings are taken in the same position for comparison, but should include one standing reading of HR.

Respirations are determined by counting the number of times the chest rises and falls in 15 seconds, then multiply by 4 to obtain the number of respirations per minute. The typical resting range is 16-20 respirations per minute; however, significant variations may be noted. Review of the medical chart should reveal the cause of variations. Guidelines for acceptable changes in respirations for dressing have not been established, however, large increases in respirations after dressing may be accompanied by the perception of shortness of breath, and may indicate the need for training in techniques to minimize the shortness of breath.

C. TIME: The amount of time required for dressing is noted, excluding the time required for the therapist to monitor vital signs, and to obtain clothing from closets (although the latter is included in evaluation of tolerance for complete A.M. care).

D. NUMBER OF REST PERIODS: The number of times the patient must stop to rest during dressing is noted.

E. SYMPTOMS: Those noted are checked.

F. BORG'S RATE OF PERCEIVED EXERTION SCALE: Use

of this scale was described by Shanfield.[11] It is used by reliable patients to self-rate perceived work effort. Improvement may be noted by a lower perceived effort for the same level of work.

G. INCORPORATION OF LABOR SAVING TECHNIQUES: Status can be noted either by spontaneous incorporation of techniques during dressing, or by the number of cues that the therapist gives the patient.

H. INCORPORATION OF BREATHING TECHNIQUES: Status is noted as above. Breathing techniques include diaphragmatic breathing, pursed lip breathing, resting positions, and coordination of inhalation/exhalation with bending and exertion. These techniques have been described by Ogden,[12] and are more beneficial for the patient with chronic obstructive pulmonary disease, although diaphragmatic breathing is frequently encouraged in symptomatic cardiac patients to control shortness of breath during Activities of Daily Living (ADL).

I. VALSALVA ON EXERTION: The Valsalva maneuver occurs when a person performs a forced exhalation against a closed glottis. It frequently occurs during maximal isometric work. In severely deconditioned patients, some aspects of ADL can result in close to maximal isometric work.[13] Prolonged Valsalva can reduce venous return to the heart, and cause significant changes in HR, heart rhythm and BP in some cardiac patients. The patient is observed for breath holding and isometric straining while donning tight garments, fastening difficult closures, or while donning socks and shoes. The patient may require instruction to exhale with exertion in order to avoid the Valsalva maneuver.

J. FUNCTIONAL WORK TOLERANCE: The total score for dressing is calculated using the functional work tolerance scale (see Figure 2). Patients with a total score of 1-5 points are considered to have good functional work tolerance for dressing; those who score between 6-14 points have fair tolerance; and those with a score greater than 15 have poor functional work tolerance. Patients with scores greater than 15 may not be candidates for some aspects of independent self care, or may require close monitoring and activity modifications to bring their score into an acceptable range.

FUNCTIONAL WORK TOLERANCE SCALE—DRESSING

Figure 2 illustrates the rating scale used to score functional work tolerance. The rating system follows.

Figure 2

BURKE REHABILITATION CENTER OCCUPATIONAL THERAPY DEPARTMENT

FUNCTIONAL WORK TOLERANCE SCALE – DRESSING

	SCORING		POINTS
COMPLETION OF ACTIVITY	Yes	0 pts	
	No	15 pts	
VITAL SIGNS	Not significant	0 pts	
	Disproportionate or prolonged recovery	2 pts	
	Significant	15 pts	
TIME	10 min or less	0 pts	
	10 – 15 min	1 pt	
	15^+ min	2 pts	
NUMBER OF REQUIRED REST PERIODS	None	0 pts	
	1 – 2	5 pts	
	3 or more	10 pts	
SYMPTOMS	Absent	0 pts	
	Mild	1 pt	
	Moderate	6 pts	
	Severe	15 pts	
ABILITY TO PERFORM SIMILAR SUCCESSIVE ACTIVITY	Yes	0 pts	
	Yes with 5 min rest	3 pts	
	No	15 pts	

KEY: Good 0 – 5 pts Fair 6 – 14 pts Poor 15 or more pts

How to Rate Activity

COMPLETION OF ACTIVITY: Score 0 points if the patient completes dressing. Score 15 points if the patient is unable to complete the activity due to EKG changes, significant changes in HR or BP, or symptoms.

VITAL SIGNS: Score 0 points if HR and BP changes stay within pre-established guidelines and return to pre-activity levels within 2 minutes of rest. Score 2 points if there is a disproportionate increase in HR and BP, or if HR or BP require longer than 2 minutes of rest to return to the pre-activity level. The 2 minute time frame was determined after several years of observation of deconditioned, complicated, or high risk cardiac patients between 10 days and 4 weeks after myocardial infarction (MI), coronary artery bypass graft (CABG), or valve surgery. Score 15 points if HR or BP exceed pre-established guidelines. General guidelines for cardiac patients up to 3 months after MI or CABG are:

HR—should not increase more than:[14]
    20 beats/min. above standing resting HR in patients post MI
    30 beats/min. above standing resting HR in patients post CABG
    —should not exceed 120 beats/min. or limits set by an exercise tolerance test[10,14]
    —should not decrease with increased workload

BP—systolic should not increase more than 20-25 mm Hg.
    —systolic should not exceed 180 mm Hg or decrease more than 20 mm Hg[10]
    —diastolic should not increase or decrease more than 10 mm Hg. and should not exceed 100-110 mm Hg or drop below 50 mm Hg[10]

The heart rate guidelines noted above were established by a survey of administrators of 31 cardiac rehabilitation programs throughout the United States, three in Canada, and one in Sweden.[14] Although these guidelines were established for exercise prescription in healthy adult patients after MI or CABG, similar guidelines are commonly used in occupational therapy ADL programs for cardiac patients.[10] The systolic blood pressure (SBP) increase guidelines are based on the assumption that dressing requires 2-2.5 times the resting oxygen consumption (METS),[4,8] and that SBP increases 7-10 mm Hg. per MET.[15] Guidelines for other types of patients should be established with the physician.

TIME: Score 0 points if dressing is completed in less than 10 minutes, score 1 point if dressing is completed in 10-15 minutes, and score 2 points if greater than 15 minutes is required for the physical act of donning clothing. This time frame was established for fairly independent patients through observation as noted previously and would need to be modified for those who require physical assistance.

NUMBER OF REQUIRED REST PERIODS: Score 0 points if dressing is completed with no rest periods to relieve symptoms or maintain vital signs within an acceptable range, score 5 points if 1-2 rests are required, score 10 points if 3 or more rests are required.

SYMPTOMS: Score 0 points for absent symptoms, score 1 point for mild symptoms, score 6 points for moderate symptoms, and score 15 points for severe symptoms. Fatigue is mild if it is relieved by up to 2 minutes of seated rest, moderate if it is relieved by 2-5 minutes of seated rest, and severe if the patient complains of exhaustion and requires bed rest or longer than 5 minutes of seated rest upon completion.

Shortness of breath is considered mild for 1+ dyspnea, moderate for 2+ dyspnea, and severe for 3+ or 4+ dyspnea using the dyspnea scale described by Ogden;[10,12] or mild for Level 1 and 2, moderate for Level 3, and severe for Level 4 in the Shortness of Breath Index described by Shanfield.[11]

Angina, sensation of pain, and dizziness are considered mild for Level 1, moderate for Level 2, and severe for Level 3 and 4 in the scale described by Ogden.[10]

ABILITY TO PERFORM SIMILAR SUCCESSIVE TASK: Score 0 points if the patient is able to perform another task at a similar energy requirement immediately upon completion of dressing. Score 3 points if up to 5 minutes rest is required, either due to symptoms or vital sign changes. Score 15 points of bedrest or longer than 5 minutes of seated rest are required.

SCORE: Add up the total number of points and assign a grade for functional work tolerance using the key (either good, fair, or poor).

SUMMARY

The monitored dressing evaluation isolates one area of self care and provides information valuable to the occupational therapist as it establishes the basis of ADL program planning for patients with low endurance. It can be used to document changes in the patient's status, and to justify the occupational therapy program. It is especially useful for the patient at a low level of function. The varibles used to score the functional work tolerance for dressing can be modified (e.g., time frame guidelines) to evaluate and document progress for other isolated activities or for a succession of ADL activities (e.g., showering, grooming, and dressing).

CONCLUSION

Successful performance of ADL is an important goal for persons with disability. For people with low endurance, the physical effort required for independent ADL may deplete their energy resources and restrict their ability to participate in other meaningful activities. Occupational therapists are the professionals most concerned with ADL, and are encountering greater numbers of patients with serious limitations. More precise ways to quantify levels of performance and change in performance can be critical components of treatment planning. Both therapists and their patients find better levels of confidence with treatment activities in which gains can be actually measured. Burke Rehabilitation Center's monitored dressing evaluation is one such tool.

REFERENCES

1. Hendrickson D, Anderson J, Gordon E: A physiological approach to the regulation of activity in the cardiac convalescent. *Am J Occup Ther* 14: 292-296, 1960
2. Gordon EE, Anderson M: Work prescription for cardiacs in the convalescent stage. *J Am Med Assoc* 183: 139-141, 1963
3. Seiser, C: Occupational therapy and cardiac rehabilitation. In *Physical Disabilities Manual*, Abreu B, Editor. New York: Raven press, 183-199, 1981
4. Ogden LD: Activity guidelines for early subacute and high risk cardiac patients. *Am J Occup Ther* 33: 291-298, 1977
5. Harrington K, Smith K, Schumacher M, Lunsford B, Watson K, Selvester R: Cardiac rehabilitation: evaluation and intervention less than 6 weeks after myocardial infarction. *Arch Phys Med Rehab* 62: 151-155, 1981
6. American Occupational Therapy Association: *Cardiac Rehabilitation,* Rockville, Md: Practice Division, 1980
7. Trombly CA, Scott AD: *Occupational Therapy for Physical Dysfunction,* Baltimore: Williams & Wilkins Co, 1980
8. Colorado heart Association: *Exercise Equivalents,* Denver, Co., p. 18
9. Ogden LD: *Procedure Guidelines for Monitored Self Care Evaluation.* Downey, CA: Cardiac Rehabilitation Resources, 1980
10. Ogden, LD: *Guidelines for Analysis and Testing of ADL with Cardiac Patients.* Downey, CA: Cardiac Rehabilitation, Inc., 1980

11. Shanfield K: Physiological monitoring: assessment of energy cost. *Occup Ther Health Care* 1: 87-97, 1984

12. Ogden LD: *Chronic Obstructive Pulmonary Disease,* Laurel, Md.: Ramsco Publishing Co., 1985

13. Haskell W: Design of a cardiac conditioning program. In *Exercise and the Heart,* Wenger NK, Editor. Philadelphia: F A Davis Company, p. 97, 1978

14. Pollock M, Ward A, Foster C: Exercise prescription for rehabilitation of the cardiac patient. In *Heart Disease and Rehabilitation,* Pollock ML and Schmidt DH, Editors. Boston: Houghton, Mifflin Professional Publishers, 413-445, 1980

15. The Committee on Exercise: *Exercise Testing and Training of Individuals with Heart Disease or at High Risk for its Development: A Handbook for Physicians.* American Heart Association, 12-13, 1975

Cardiac Rehabilitation: Low Energy Considerations

Karen Bird, OTR/L
Scott Phelps, OTR/L

ABSTRACT. Occupational therapy plays a significant role in helping patients with coronary artery disease move to restored health and function and in facilitating their change from states of crisis to adaptation. Treatment begun early and carried out both in group and individual sessions, addresses cardiac function and risk factors in all phases of daily activities with emphasis on managing stress. Activities of daily living groups particularly emphasize energy conservation techniques in both vocational and avocational pursuits. Staff also teach and encourage appropriate life style modifications.

St. Vincent Charity Hospital and Health Center (SVCH&HC) is a 400 bed acute care Catholic institution operated by the Sisters of Charity of St. Augustine. Located in downtown Cleveland, Ohio, it offers services to the entire lakeshore area of Ohio. A cardiac rehabilitation program was developed by the Occupational Therapy Department to fit within a multi-disciplinary team philosophy and aimed at restoring patients with cardiac disability to maximum physical, psychosocial and vocational status. The primary objective of the program is to help the person with a cardiac condition, and his family prepare for making alterations in living patterns that could reduce the risk of recurrence of heart attack.

Heart attack is the number one killer in the United States, affecting

Both Karen Nicole Bird and Scott Phelps are staff therapists at St. Vincent Charity Hospital and Health Center in Cleveland, OH. Ms. Bird has functioned as staff therapist, currently specializing in cardiac rehabilitation and substance abuse. She has also performed duties in psychiatry and supervision. She is currently completing the requirements for a Master's Degree in Human Services at John Carroll University. Mr. Phelps has been working largely in the area of physical disabilities, hand rehabilitation, NDT and in pulmonary rehabilitation.

This article appears jointly in *Occupational Therapy for the Energy Deficient Patient* (The Haworth Press, 1986) and *Occupational Therapy in Health Care*, Volume 3, Number 1 (Spring 1986).

more than one million Americans annually. Modern scientific research and technology have refined medical treatment and enhanced pharmaceutical intervention to help individuals survive initial acute cardiac problems. However, lifestyle modifications are imperative to survival in prevention of potentially fatal reoccurrences. The individual quickly and sometimes hesistantly learns that adjustments in their activities of daily living is of utmost importance. The "cardiac cripple" patient will be fearful and live accordingly—unable to perform the simplest of activities. Other individuals will seek courageously and positively the formidable task of directly confronting their disease with the goal of "moving forward". This paper will address the cardiac rehabilitation program created by St. Vincent Charity Hospital (SVCH) to help persons survive cardiac episodes and 'get on with life', and will describe the rationale for its development and its activities which focus particularly on anxiety and its effect on energy depletion.

OCCUPATIONAL THERAPY CARDIAC REHABILITATION

As an acute hospital in an urban area, St. Vincent has a large population of patients with cardiac disease. Because persons are so seriously affected, both physically and psychologically, by heart attack and are therefore often 'disabled' in the activities of their daily lives, the occupational therapy staff wished to develop a program that would focus on reducing this disability, enabling patients to resume as normal lives as possible.

The program was developed to be conducted in three phases, extending over an average of two weeks to two years. It includes both restorative and maintenance components (graded activity and education) and attempts to match each persons regime to his own habit structure and life style. Phase I begins when the patient is admitted to the hospital with the heart attack, or 7 to 10 days after cardiac surgery. Programming begins immediately with education and counseling regarding heart function and its relationship to daily activities. This is done either one to one or in a group environment depending on the patient's status. Classes/treatment sessions focus on stress management and/or energy conservation. Throughout hospitalization the patient attends such sessions where he is helped to apply the principles to his own habit structure and daily routines.

As soon as the patient is discharged, Phase II begins and is carried out on an outpatient basis from then on, giving specific attention to each individual's needs and problems/questions as they adjust to home environments. Phase III is an extension of Phase II and is conducted through classes arranged by the cardiac rehabilitation team and conducted by various staff members (occupational therapists, dietitians, exercise technicians, and nursing personnel.) Patients attend according to interest and need but are encouraged to attend all sessions. The class series takes twelve weeks usually. Class topics include:

1. Stress Management I
2. Stress Management II
3. Leisure and CAD (Coronary Artery Disease)
4. Anatomy and CAD
5. Risk Factors of CAD
6. You, Cholesterol and Your Heart
7. You and Your Medications
8. Sodium and Your Heart I
9. Sodium and Your Heart II
10. Decision Making
11. Value of Exercise
12. Focus Ahead I
13. Focus Ahead II
14. Tobacco and CAD
15. Energy Conservation as it Relates to your Work and Home Environment
16. Time Management
17. Communicating Effectively

All three phases of the program are designed to offer support for return to fitness as well as for maintenance of individual productivity. The group process involved, as persons are adjusting to new ways of thinking about their daily activities, is a strong component of the program.

EMPHASIS ON PSYCHOSOCIAL FACTORS

In occupational therapy after initial evaluation, which includes history taking, chart reviews, interviews with the patient and his/her family, checklists to identify interests, life style and team meetings, primary goals of treatment are the establishment of good rapport with the patient and diminishment of his anxiety.He needs to have confidence that staff understand and appreciate his concerns and personal expectations. The major psychological needs at this time for the patient with coronary artery disease are to resolve feelings of anxiety and depression. The occupational therapy program attends to both these feelings in definite ways.

How and why patients reach states of arousal and anxiety vary widely; therefore evaluating anxiety patterns in each individual is of utmost importance in order to choose and grade program activities appropriately. The anxiety response in patients with CAD is based on two major feelings, helplessness and the threat of death. Anxiety when evaluated is therefore classified by levels to guide treatment:

1. Mild (behavior—increased alertness)
2. Moderate (behavior—decreased alertness, decreased acuity of hearing and vision)
3. Severe (behavior—decreased thought processes and impaired ability to make decisions)
4. Panic (behavior—complete disassociation in thought [rare in CAD patients])[1 p76]

There are three major components of anxiety which can be observed during the evaluation and treatment process. They are: (1) appearance, (2) behavior, (3) conversation. Some examples of physical reactions of anxious patients are as follows: increased restlessness, decreased fine motor control, pallor, increased pulse rate and respiration. Examples of psychosocial responses related to anxiety include many somatic complaints "I feel pain in my right arm", "My teeth hurt", etc. In addition they may project feelings of self through statements such as "My family is worried that I am going to die", "My supervisor thinks that I won't be able to do my job at work". Anxiety can keep the CAD patient from concentrating, from making decisions, or taking control of his life. Previous values and goals may change and energy will be directed simply to restoring physical functioning. The therapist must be able to identify these signs and evaluate levels of anxiety accurately.

Coping mechanisms are important to recognize as the patient adjusts to his perceived disability. As used by patients with cardiac disease coping style falls into two major categories:[1 p105]

1. Problems are eliminated through denial, disbelief or repression
2. Loss of function or disability is rationalized or intellectualized.

Hospital personnel frequently think that patients of category #2 understand and integrate information and medical instructions better than patients of category #1. This is not necessarily true, however, as anxiety manifests itself in many ways that can disguise actual feelings. Accordingly, a concept to remember in planning treatment for persons with cardiac disease is that *all* defense mechanisms are initially pertinent for survival and give the patient both motivation and 'energy' to live. In view of this, the philosophy of treatment at SVCH is based on helping each person restore human dignity through control over activities of daily living. In addition, it involves helping the patient to be aware of his rehabilitation potentials, to move as needed through the 'Six Stages of Grieving' (for depression)[2] and to give support and show awareness to individual concerns through application of principles of Maslow's hierarchy of needs in program design.

EMPHASIS ON PHYSICAL LIMITATIONS

Myocardial infarction (MI) represents a physical insult to the heart which affects its tissues and their ability to contract. Since the heart is a muscle which demands oxygen to meet various needs, depending on performance level, when a portion of the heart is denied oxygen, pain occurs and possibly some of the heart tissue dies. When this happens an MI has occurred and this muscle death permanently affects the efficiency of the heart muscle. The extent of difficulty is based both on the severity of the infarct and its location. Generally, in an 'uncomplicated' MI, most patients have decreased efficiency of heart output which in turn causes a decrease in energy. This loss of heart performance is characterized by pain and dysrhythmia attributed to the MI and can be intensified by environmental factors such as extremes of temperature, air pollution, altitude and stress, as well as by excess levels of activity.[1]

The occupational therapy program for these patients therefore, through its educational components, assists patients, understanding of their condition by reviewing heart function and the rationale behind rating and limiting activities, as well as learning the affects of exposure to adverse environmental conditions.

For example, patients are taught that excessive heat and humidity hamper body cooling efforts. Under such conditions blood vessels dilate to increase the peripheral circulation to promote cooling. This decreases central core blood volume and stroke volume with each heart beat. The heart rate, therefore, must increase to meet O_2 requirements and that puts increased demands on the heart.[4] Patients are helped to see that they can lower the demands on their hearts in hot weather by limiting activity. Cold temperatures, on the other hand, cause increased vasoconstriction and thereby can produce negative effects on the heart. Since increase in vasoconstriction increases peripheral vascular resistance, arterial blood pressure rises, resulting in greater O_2 demands.[1] Quality of the atmosphere is also significant. That is why 'air alerts' are now so common in cities and why persons with cardiac problems need to attend to activity levels when air pollution is bad.

Since all activities put increased demands on the heart, patients must learn it is the *level* of the demand of a given activity and the response of the heart that are of concern. If demands are too great or come too soon after an MI, pain or dysrhythmias may occur inhibiting the recovery process.

In the SVCH cardiac rehabilitation program, occupational therapy includes an educational emphasis to help patients cope with their limited energy levels created by decreased efficiency of the heart. Patients are introduced to work simplification principles, to efficient energy use, to stress management techniques and to leisure counseling all to control their efforts and the demands placed on their hearts. Patients are introduced to these concepts through discussions and teaching materials and, as appropriate, based on their stage of recovery and progress, may be placed in situations to apply techniques and principles learned. This educational process is usually group oriented and is often also video-taped to be available for review and discussion with staff as well as with fellow patients. Activities chosen can be those that match individual patient's and/or the groups interests and needs.

Work simplification principles are stressed and patients are helped to analyze their various ADL tasks and/or employment responsibilities to choose ways of performing that maximize the flow of work and minimize the effort and stress on the heart. Specific applications may include tool modifications, use of particular body mechanics, adjustment of working positions and/or use of energy-saving equipment.

Leisure activities are valuable in promoting a sense of enjoyment and self worth. They are also very gradable in terms of the energy demand and may be a good precursor to work. Leisure counselling is therefore used to address the activity levels of these avocational activities. The therapist assists in helping the patient maximize the benefits of leisure and minimize the threat of overexertion.

In order to help patients think about and plan activities to maximize their available energy, the occupational therapy program spends much time on activity pacing, that is, the mixing and balancing of demanding tasks and rest, proper positioning of equipment involved in any activity and use of proper body mechanics. The MET system is a method for categorizing activities by the energy required to perform them, and is useful in helping patients plan their activity patterns. As used at SVCH a patient who has had an MI is introduced to the rating of activities according to O_2 demand and is then instructed to begin his recovery with activities demanding the least amounts of energy. As recovery progresses, activities demanding more energy may be incorporated into daily schedules. The rate of progression of activity is determined by the physician based on severity of the MI, the patient's level of compliance and the patient's response to activity. Activities or tasks are adjusted to require different METs, thereby facilitating recovery or providing guidelines to the patient as to which activities are or are not feasible at his stage of recovery. This physical component of the occupational therapy program is carefully monitored and is equally important and must co-exist with the psychosocial emphasis in a cardiac rehabilitation regime. Each patient's needs must be determined individually and treatment must be designed and graded to facilitate safe and active return to the productive living that is satisfying to each individual.

SUMMARY

The cardiac rehabilitation program in occupational therapy at SVCH has been described, illustrating the shared emphasis on psychosocial adjustment as well as physical restoration. These goals are achieved through an educational and counseling approach that attends to each individual's pre-morbid life style and interests as well as his current and anticipated cardiac status. Through careful teaching of principles of work simplification, energy conservation, and coping mechanisms patients learn through practice, safe and active return to daily activities.

CONCLUSION

The occupational therapy program described is an example of how immediate intervention with persons who have coronary artery disease can facilitate energy gain and return to satisfying daily function in an illness in which psychosocial and physical energy loss is dramatic. Restoration of control over one's life style through teaching how to plan and engage in one's activities of daily living is coupled with assisting the patient to gain hope; thus he learns to 'harness' his free floating anxiety and return sooner to an optimal state of performance.

ADDENDUM

Various evaluations and teaching materials are used by the therapists in the Cardiac Rehabilitation Program. They include: A Life Change Scale, Behavior Pattern Questionnaire, Symptoms Checklist, Burnout Checklist and Scale as well as materials related to Stress Management and Energy Conservation. Persons who are interested in knowing more about any or all of these items should contact the authors at:

Occupational Therapy Department
St. Vincent Charity Hospital & Health Center
2351 E. 22nd Street
Cleveland, OH 44122

REFERENCES

1. Cornett, Sandra J.; Watson, Joan E. *Cardiac Rehabilitation An Interdisciplinary Team Approach,* 1984. John Wiley & Sons, Inc.
2. Kubler-Ross. *On Death and Dying,* 1969. MacMillan Publishing Company
3. Trombly, Catherine A. *Occupational Therapy for Physical Dysfunction,* 1977
4. Rowell, L.B.; Marz, H.J.; Bruce, R.A., et al. Reductions in cardiac output, central blood volume and stroke volume with thermal stress in normal men during exercise. *Journal of Clinical Investigation,* 1966, 45, 1801-1816

ADDITIONAL REFERENCES

A. Davis, Martha; McKay, Matthew; Eshelman, Elizabeth. *The Relaxation and Stress Reduction Workbook,* 1982. New Harbinger Publications
B. St. Vincent Charity Hospital & Health Center. *Cardiac Rehabilitation Booklet,* 1985

PRACTICE WATCH:
THINGS TO THINK ABOUT

Adapting to Life After a Stroke:
A Personal Account of One Patient's
Physical and Psychological
Problem-Solving Efforts

Susan P. Lindheim

ABSTRACT. This article provides a patient's perspective on the physical and psychological adaptations necessitated by a stroke. The subject of the article is 70 year old woman who has suffered two severe strokes. Her efforts in adapting to energy deficits and relearning how to walk, write, speak, carry out the activities of daily living, and resume her exercise program are all detailed. In addition, the psychological adaptions that she has made in order to cope with the strokes are described. The subject's extremely positive attitude and determination are highlighted, along with her perceptions of how therapists can help other people who have had strokes develop a similar positive attitude.

In Greek mythology, the character Sisyphus was doomed to roll a stone up a hill. But every time he got near the top, the stone would roll back down to the bottom and he would have to start his struggle

Susan Lindheim, the granddaughter of the subject of this paper, is at the time of writing a junior at Beverly Hills High School, Beverly Hills, CA, where she is actively involved in journalism classes and activities.

This article appears jointly in *Occupational Therapy for the Energy Deficient Patient* (The Haworth Press, 1986) and *Occupational Therapy in Health Care*, Volume 3, Number 1 (Spring 1986).

again, never to succeed. Thus Pearl Lindheim, survivor of two strokes and now a leader of stroke therapy classes, describes the mental anguish that strokes can bring. "Every time you think you're rising above a certain level, the littlest thing breaks you down and you sink to the bottom and you have to start all over again to get up."

Pearl is not atypical in her experience adapting to her strokes. Her rechanneling of her energy to meet her new needs is not unusual. However, what distinguishes Pearl Lindheim is her attitude, determination and strong will to live a fulfilled life. As a survivor of two strokes she feels reborn, refreshed, renewed. She views her strokes not as a horrible problem to be painfully overcome, but rather as an opportunity to reflect upon her life and to discover new things, ideas and people that she might not otherwise have met. And Pearl refuses to be told that she cannot do something. She can and she will, making her a paragon for others.

TWO STROKES AND THEIR AFTERMATHS

Pearl had been very active for all of her life before her first stroke. She had total family-care responsibility for a large home and its many occupants: two sons, her husband, her parents, and her grandmother. In addition, she assumed sole responsibility for the wellbeing of various other aged relatives who lived alone and required almost constant attention. For thirty five years she also played golf twice a week, often competing in tournaments and winning many prizes. Her community activities included her work as a hospital volunteer, working one day a week in the ophthamology department of a large public institution. Her two strokes, however, changed all of this.

What began as vague, flu-like symptoms one weekend in December 1978 soon turned into complete paralysis and an inability to speak. Pearl drifted in and out of consciousness for weeks, during which time her doctors predicted that she would not live. But this only made Pearl more determined. "Who was he (the doctor) to tell me whether I was going to live or not? I refused to say that anybody but God can take my life or judge whether I'm going to live or not."

Pearl was to recover from this stroke only to suffer another two and one-half years later. This one, even more devastating for Pearl, left her partially paralyzed on her right side. She is receiving therapy in order to recover completely from this stroke, and although she has recovered somewhat, she still has only partial movement in her right arm and moves her right leg only with difficulty.

BASIC ADAPTATIONS:
RELEARNING HOW TO SPEAK, WRITE AND WALK

After Pearl's first stroke, everything changed; her entire high energy lifestyle was molded toward a determined recovery. Pearl lost her speech with the first stroke, so her first step on the arduous road to recovery was relearning how to speak. Her voice was slurred and she had to work hard to regain complete control of her communication. Even now, she comments, at times it feels as if her tongue is a heavy whale inside her mouth and she has to make a concerted effort to speak clearly. And she does have word recall difficulties.

Then Pearl had to relearn how to write. She could no longer hold a pencil, and she tried to adapt. She learned to print first, practicing every day by writing her name. Her husband, Gilbert, would dictate sentences to her for an hour each day, simple sentences, until she learned to write again.

Walking was the next step toward recovery. Gradually she learned to move her legs. Then she walked with a walker until she had made enough progress to advance to a heavy, cumbersome three-pronged cane. She would work constantly, three to four hours a day, to recover. She lifted weights on her leg, sometimes as much as 15 pounds, twice daily. She says that it was exhausting work. "But I programmed myself that I had to do these things in order to survive and be a person again and be able to handle myself."

Throughout Pearl's recovery the therapists told her that she could not do things, and she would then prove them wrong. They said she would never walk and now she can walk without dependence on a cane. Their negativity made her more determined. She programmed herself for success. "I feel that it's not up to a therapist or doctor to tell you what you can do. What you can do is up to you as a person. *You* have to be the one to decide what you can do. Once you take a defeatist attitude you're gone completely."

Pearl admits that, although she has an active life, she does, at times, become very tired. She explains that even the simplest tasks consume twice as much of her energy as they would of a person who has not had a stroke.

ADL ADAPTATIONS:
BATHING, DRESSING, COOKING, DRIVING

One problem Pearl faced in adapting to life after her stroke was dressing and bathing. Because one leg is still partially paralyzed, to dress she must lay out all her clothes around where she will dress. She then sits down and puts on her clothes, rising only after she is completely dressed. To shower, she first puts her towel and cane over the towel rack on the wall. She then places a bath chair in the shower and puts the mat down. She stands to wash her upper body, but sits down to wash her legs. Then, to get out, she pulls the towel off the rack to dry herself and then uses her cane to leave the shower.

Pearl also had to modify her activities in the kitchen in order to adapt. She had to learn new ways of balancing her partially paralyzed body, just as she had to discover the most efficient movements in the kitchen. For instance, in order to put a pot filled with water on the stove, she must first place the empty pot on the stove, since she cannot carry a full pot and her cane. She then brings over a bottle of water to fill the pot.

Driving was also a problem. "The first time I got in the car, it was absolutely frightening, like I'd never driven before." Pearl was frightened by the movement. Slowly she began to remember how to drive and she practiced around several blocks until she regained her confidence. After the second stroke she had to adapt her method of driving because her right leg was not strong or quick enough to move from the gas to the brake. Therefore she now uses two legs for driving: her right leg for the gas, as she can move it up and down quickly enough to get to the gas, and her left leg for the brake.

RESUMING PHYSICAL ACTIVITIES

Pearl has now resumed some of her physical activities since her strokes. Always an active person, she refused to let low energy be an excuse for inactivity. She rides an exercise bicycle twice a day for four to five miles each day as therapy for her weakened leg. She throws balls in her yard and hits golf balls to exercise her arm. And she has resumed her golf games, playing nine holes with the use of a cart. She has modified her actions to play golf. She uses the clubs as a cane, when going from the cart to the hole, and she keeps her feet farther apart when she swings so that she can keep her balance.

Swimming has always been a part of Pearl's life, and she is not handicapped in the water. But getting into the pool required adaptations. To get in, she holds onto the rail and lowers herself down the steps into the pool fairly easily. But she cannot use the stair rail alone to pull herself out along the stairway because her one free arm is not strong enough to help lift her leg. To get out she needs some assistance.

PSYCHOLOGICAL ADAPTATIONS

More trying than the physical adaptations to her stroke were the psychological problems that Pearl faced as she found herself dependent to a much greater extent on her husband and on others for such taxing physical activities as traveling, large scale marketing, and clothes shopping. "Dependency is so devastating after you've been in complete control and you find yourself unable to handle your problems and your tasks." Dependency, she says, causes a great loss of self esteem. And this is then harder to surmount than the physical handicaps created by the stroke.

To adapt to her stroke psychologically, Pearl has rechanneled her energy. She goes to school to learn about new subjects. "I made up my mind that the stroke wasn't going to devastate me. As long as I had my mind, I was going to use it."

Pearl also wanted to help others, and she therefore joined a stroke foundation where she leads a group of stroke victims, counseling them with understanding. From this experience she has learned much, and her classes have also benefitted. She says that some days stroke patients feel very shaky, and that they can cry very easily. "The mere fact that I walk into there so confident that life is good and worth living has helped many of them."

What has also helped Pearl surmount the depression that strokes can bring is the support of her husband. He gives her self esteem and he gives her hope. "He never says I can't do something. He always says, 'You can. Try.' "

A PATIENT'S PERSPECTIVE

Pearl's advice to other stroke victims is to get interested in something to rechannel whatever energy they have to become involved in something new instead of just feeling sorry for themselves. "Use this time of your life to learn something. Learning is the greatest test of your ability to live."

She says that strokes cause a loss of self esteem which first manifests itself as anger at yourself and at the world. Then this anger becomes depression. But victims should not allow themselves to become depressed. "The depression can ruin you before you start." Rather they should view their stroke as a puzzle that they must solve. Patients should also associate with other people instead of being ashamed of their handicaps.

Her advice to therapists is not to treat their patients like objects. Such treatment only causes the patients to feel like objects, which is very detrimental to their self esteem. She also advises therapists to beware of baby talk. Too many people approach handicapped persons as if they were small children, causing great harm. "After all," she says, "metamorphosis does not set in. You are still the same human being that you were before the stroke. The only changes are a physical handicap."

Therapists, she says, should not belittle their patients by talking down to them. Rather they should say, "It's up to you. It's all in your hands and if you do it and you're conscientious, you will make progress." Therapists should also not be negative. Rather they should give positive support. "Nobody can say how far you can go. Even a therapist can't tell you exactly. It's up to *you.*"

CONCLUSION

Sisyphus found no joy in his task; he found only weary frustration. At times Pearl, as a result of her strokes, feels tired and deterred. But she does not give in; she does not allow herself to fall into despair. Rather, Pearl's frustrations only strengthen her determination. She sees obstacles not as negative problems but rather as positive learning experiences. She has developed a strong will to survive and to help others lead satisfying lives. Her attitude has made her different. And though she may feel down at times, she will never succumb to Sisyphus' miserable fate.

SOMETHING NEW AND USEFUL . . .

Creation of ''All About Aging'': A Simulation Board Game

Ferol Menks, MS, OTR

The idea for this game was conceived when the author attended a workshop by the National Medical Audiovisual Clearinghouse at the University of Florida on simulation and gaming for health professionals. As an occupational therapy educator she was interested in learning additional teaching strategies. She decided to create a game that could be used in the course in human growth and development that she was teaching at the University of Florida. ''I was very concerned that the students I was teaching, who were mainly between 19 and 21 years of age, did not understand very much about what it felt like to be old. They were limited in their knowledge concerning the elderly to what they learned from their grandparents or persons that they may have encountered in nursing homes. Their exposure to a wide cross section of the elderly was very limited.''

''The Road of Life'' was created to facilitate students' affective learning of some of the common physical and psychosocial experiences common among the elderly. Of the many simulation games on aging, none was available that was short, simple, and required the players to experience handicaps, as well as physical and psychosocial events. She wanted to develop something that was

This article appears jointly in *Occupational Therapy for the Energy Deficient Patient* (The Haworth Press, 1986) and *Occupational Therapy in Health Care*, Volume 3, Number 1 (Spring 1986).

115

educational and would provide affective learning experiences and also be fun.

The author reviewed the literature and interviewed older persons. She asked them, "What makes you happy? What makes you sad? Tell me about several things that happened to you and your friends lately. What makes life worthwhile for you now?" From these sources and from her experience in working with the elderly, game cards were created. These were continually refined over a period of 3 years to provide realistic experiences that were frequently encountered among the elderly. Gains and losses in terms of life units were assigned. "I was very concerned that the game not be depressing and reinforce negative attitudes about the elderly. It took alot of field testing and refining to be sure that this did not happen."

The game was born and was first played with students in a course in growth and development at the University of Florida. The game board was hand drawn on mat board and the game equipment and bag handmade. The students responded very favorably to the game. The author then decided to present it at the National Association for Simulation and Gaming Conference. The handmade game board was professionally done by the Learning Resource Center and nicer fabric was used for the homemade game bags. This was the authors' first presentation at a conference. When she arrived, some very sophisticated games were being presented. The Army had simulations of the world and wars and battles. The political scientists had intricate and elaborate games. "It was very scary and I expected to have no one attend my presentation. However, the room was overflowing and the response was very positive." Some excellent suggestions were provided and revisions and fine tuning were again done. People kept requesting to borrow the game and a form was developed for people to complete when they played the game so that this would provide valuable field testing information. Over 600 persons responded to the questionnaires. Persons from a variety of settings and backgrounds kept asking to borrow the game such as 4H leaders, church groups, rehabilitation centers, psychologists, other educators in a variety of disciplines, occupational therapists, etc. Its use and applicability seemed to expand beyond what its creator originally foresaw. "The game seemed to have a life of its own."

The author presented the game at the American Occupational Therapy Association Annual Conference and the response was again very positive. People kept asking for the game and her homemade copies needed to give way to publishing it in order to make it available to those who wanted copies. The task of finding a publisher was one that took tenacity and endurance. Over one hundred publishers were contacted and one was interested. The University of Florida and Ferol Menks entered into an agreement about copyright and division of royalties. Nurseco, Inc., began preparations to publish it. Two years later the game was finally published and available. Some more revisions were made. The title was changed to "All About Aging" since Milton Bradley, Inc., who did not want to publish the game, wrote that the title was too close to their "Game of Life". Nurseco, Inc. was soon after this purchased by Williams and Wilkins, Inc.

The whole process has been a real learning experience. This author now understands what writers mean when they talk about the characters creating the story and having their own life. What happens seems to come from the creation itself.

A Preliminary Critique

All About Aging—A Simulation Board Game, designed by Ferol Menks, MS, OTR. Distributed by Williams and Wilkins, 428 E. Preston St., Baltimore, MD 21202. Price: $25.95

Note: The following review is based on trial use of the game by occupational therapy personnel with patients in a nursing home. Further exploration of its potential will be conducted with other groups and settings.

The content of the game is excellent for the purposes of training staff of convalescent hospitals, residential care facilities, for volunteers who provide services to the elderly and other groups who have interest in the aging process.

In this evaluation the game was played by ten adults with various physical handicaps and three members of the professional staff. Their comments were as follows:

1. Instructions do not specify that the red chips are the life units.
2. The red chips are difficult to pick up. This would be a particular problem if the game were to be used by sensorially impaired persons.
3. Directional arrows on the board are somewhat confusing.
4. Adaptation for either a short or long version would be an advantage when using the game for in-service training.
5. The price seems excessive for what is provided.
6. A Life Preserve Box is mentioned, but is not clearly identified.
7. The game is fun and has the potential for improving sensitivity to the problems of aging.

Ardith D. Breton, MA, OTR
Professional Consultant
Salinas, CA 93906